Marriage Reduction
and Fertility

Marriage Reduction and Fertility

David Yaukey
University of Massachusetts,
Amherst

Lexington Books
D.C. Heath and Company
Lexington, Massachusetts
Toronto   London

Duty
Davis
16 July 78

Library of Congress Cataloging in Publication Data

Yaukey, David.
    Marriage reduction and fertility.

    Includes bibliographical references.
    1. Fertility, Human. 2. Marriage. 3. Family size. I. Title.
HB903.F4Y32   3-1.32'1   73-6994
ISBN 0-669-89441-9

Copyright © 1973 by D.C. Heath and Company.

Published simultaneously in Canada.

Printed in the United States of America.

International Standard Book Number: 0-669-89441-9

Library of Congress Catalog Card Number: 73-6994

Contents

List of Figures

List of Tables

Acknowledgments

This book was written in the seclusion of my study at home in Amherst, Mass. For that ideal thinking environment, I am grateful to the University of Massachusetts for supplying me a sabbatical leave, to my colleagues in the Department of Sociology for heeding my plea to be left alone, and to my wife Barbara for tolerating the invasion of her home's privacy by a preoccupied and restless writer for several months.

I also am indebted to some of the same people for their attention when I needed it. My wife Barbara, Edwin Driver, Michael Lewis, and Etienne Van de Walle all read the first draft carefully and gave invaluable comments from their various perspectives. I hope they see an improved work as a result of their labors.

Marriage Reduction
and Fertility

1 Introduction

The arithmetic of world population growth is simple and frightening. Indeed, it is so simple and frightening that national public attention can be expected to focus on it for short periods in morbid fascination and then to swing away to other more recent popular causes. This happened with the zero-population-growth movement around 1970, and we can expect it to happen again over the decades ahead. Meanwhile, the consequences of rapid population growth will persist and increase, irrespective of public attention to them.

The role of science, in the presence of fickle public concern, is to be ready with usable knowledge when the public does become concerned. The record of demography is good in this respect, I believe. For decades before the population explosion became a subject of general alarm, demographers had been developing theory which would enable the nondemographer to comprehend those events and to see where policies could be focused. And, I submit, it behooves demographers, and other scientists concerned with population problems, to prepare to play that same role in the future.

I am convinced that sooner or later nations will contemplate in desperation the advisability of changing societal marital patterns in order to reduce rates of population growth. Policymakers and their scientist advisors may disagree among themselves as to the adequacy of voluntary family-planning programs as a *first* step in world population control.[1] But they are less and less likely to disagree in the future about the inadequacy of such a limited policy. If there is no retreat from recently won gains against mortality, and if couples continue to want more than the number of children that collectively would balance those low death rates, then eventually something has to give, for the world is finite. I believe that it is the motivation for having children which will then become the focus of attention by policymakers, and that policymakers then will contemplate changing marital patterns in order to reduce the motivation for having many children, much as Davis already has suggested.[2]

The purpose of this book is to summarize and to integrate what

1

we now know or believe about the relationship between marital patterns as a cause and fertility as an effect. It serves this purpose by providing and then elaborating a conceptual framework in which to place our scattered knowledge. That elaboration itself helps to bring hidden implications to the foreground.

But that same focus on conceptualization detracts from the adequacy of the book for other purposes. The reader who seeks exhaustive empirical verification for all of the implications suggested will be disappointed. Our use of available statistical data will be primarily for purposes of example and illustration, not for proof. Verification, and the modification of the model which surely will follow any attempts at verification, is a task beyond the scope of this short book.

This book is written both for demographers and for sociologists—particular family sociologists—interested in population problems. Although I hope for other readers as well, I am concerned that they might misconstrue my intentions or tone. The style will be intentionally detached, even when I am spelling out policy implications of some of the theory. This does not signify advocacy nor acceptance of contemplated policies such as increased divorce.[3] Rather it expresses my determination to look coldly at the population consequences of any such marital trend as part of the information necessary for considering a marriage-reduction policy.

Precursors of this Book

We have an especial debt to three bodies of thought and inquiry on our topic. First, Indian demographers have been debating from the 1960s the pros and cons of reducing their country's high birth rate by delaying age of women at first marriage.[4] Second, Kingsley Davis and Judith Blake, in the late 1960s, proposed, in spirited debate with other demographers, that changes in marital patterns might be necessary to supplement family-planning policies, not only in the long run but also in the short run.[5] Finally, demographers studying the demographic transition in Europe, Ansley Coale and Norman Ryder prominent among them, have begun to detail the role of marital changes in the fertility transition.[6] This last effort still is very much alive and indeed supplied many of the articles summarized and integrated in our book.

This book comes at a time when research relevant to the topic has begun appearing in some profusion in the learned journals. Thus, in a sense, it is opportunistic of me to pick the brains of other scholars and beat them to publication in book form. However, I write the book now out of conviction that a theoretical integration at this early stage will add to the understandability and value of the facts being produced. Moreover, I am under no illusion that this book will preempt the field. Other books on the topic already are planned, for instance by the Coale team. And, hopefully, others will be provoked by the present book.

Structure of the Book

I have attempted in this book to follow my own advice on how to theorize about fertility.[7] An earlier article distinguished among three classes of variables: fertility itself (Class C), the Davis-Blake "intermediate variables" (Class B), and the subclasses of factors identified by Ronald Freedman as influencing the Davis-Blake variables (Class A).[8] My recommendation was a strategy of focusing separately on the relations between Class A and Class B variables on the one hand, and between Class B and Class C variables on the other. In the present case, this means focusing on the relationship between marital patterns (one of the Class B variables on the Davis-Blake list) and fertility.

The immediate result of this attempt, however, was to raise a perplexing question: do marital patterns logically belong on the Davis-Blake list of "intermediate variables?" Indeed, I argue in Chapter 3, marital variables seem to fall more logically into Class A than into Class B. Accordingly, we adopt a *modification* of the Davis-Blake list in detailing the relationships between marital patterns and fertility.

The sequence of our attention dictates the sequence of treatment in the book. We start with the dependent variable (period fertility) and work backward to marital events (first marriage, marital dissolution, remarriage) as independent variables.

We break the journey into several smaller steps. In Chapter 2 we treat the relationship between period fertility and cohort fertility, thus adopting the cohort frame of reference we will employ in subsequent chapters. In Chapter 3 we treat the relationship between cohort fertility and cohort marital status, modifying the Davis-Blake framework to facilitate the treatment of that question. Chapter 4 is a tangent on illegitimacy suggested by our thinking in Chapter 3. Chapters 5 and 6 treat cohort marital status as a dependent variable and the marital events as independent variables, Chapter 5 focusing on marital dissolution and remarriage and Chapter 6 dealing with first marriage.

In Chapter 7 we try to spell out the policy implications of the substantive points made in earlier chapters. They surprised me. Perhaps they will surprise the reader as well.

2

Period Fertility and Cohort Fertility

Now we begin working back along the chain of causation from period fertility to cohort fertility, to cohort marital status, then finally to cohort marital events. The present chapter is devoted to the first link of the chain, that between period fertility and cohort fertility.

Preliminary to all, let us devote the initial section of the chapter to a conceptual review of period fertility and cohort fertility. This may seem elementary to readers who are demographers, but it should be helpful background to others.

Period Fertility and Cohort Fertility Contrasted: A Review

Fertility, as demographers use the term, refers to the actual bearing of children, not to the capacity to bear children.[a] Normally we measure the fertility of an aggregate of people by constructing a ratio. The denominator of the ratio is the number of people whose fertility performance we are measuring; the numerator is the number of births attributed to those people. The question is which people to group together in the denominator and, accordingly, which births to include in the numerator.

The two bases for aggregation being compared are the *cohort* basis and the *period* basis. These both can be seen by referring to Figure 2-1, a population pyramid. Our population pyramid is a "toy" one, referring to country X according to its census of December 31, 1900. It represents a percentage distribution of the population on the basis of sex and age. The length of the bars to the left indicate the percentage of the total population falling into each of the male age classes; the same applies for the female bars extending to the right. Unlike the presentation of most population pyramids, ours not only

---

[a]The capacity to bear children is termed *fecundity* conventionally. United Nations, *Multilingual Demographic Dictionary*, English Section (Population Studies No. 29, New York: United Nations, 1958), p. 38.

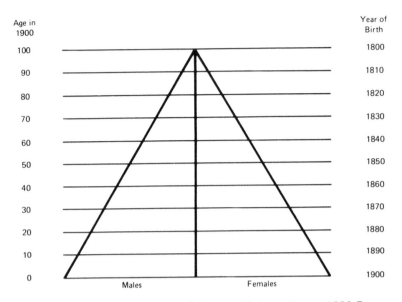

Age in
1900

Year of
Birth

100 — 1800
90 — 1810
80 — 1820
70 — 1830
60 — 1840
50 — 1850
40 — 1860
30 — 1870
20 — 1880
10 — 1890
0 — 1900

Males   Females

Figure 2-1. Population Pyramid of Country X According to 1900 Census

specifies the years of age in the left-hand margin, but also translates those years of age into the dates of birth, shown in the right-hand margin.

Thus, for instance, people who were sixty years old at the time of the 1900 census can be inferred to have been born in 1840. Collectively, these people would be referred to as the *birth cohort* of 1840.[b,c]

Suppose that, in the census of 1900, each of the sixty-year-old women was asked how many live births she had produced in her lifetime. Then we could aggregate the number of women in the cohort in the denominator and the number of live births reported by

---

[b]The demographic concept of *cohort* generally refers to people aggregated on the basis of a specified event having happened to them all at the same time. Thus one can identify marriage cohorts, divorce cohorts, and even immigration cohorts. If the term is used without further specification, assume that the demographer means a *birth cohort*, as do we.

[c]Strictly speaking, the people aged sixty in 1900 are not exactly the birth cohort of 1840. For one thing, they are only the survivors of the mortality which depleted the cohort during that sixty-year period. For another thing, the birth cohort might have lost some members through emigration. It also could have gained some through immigration, unless we limit the population to those born in country X.

them in the numerator and have a measure of *cohort completed fertility* for the survivors of the cohort.[d]

Suppose that, in that census, each of the sixty-year-old women also was asked how old she was at each of the births she mentioned. We then could construct a measure to summarize another important aspect of cohort-fertility performance, the timing of the births. For instance, we could compute an average, such as an arithmetic mean, of the reported ages of the women at the times of their childbearing: the mean *age at childbearing*.

Let us contrast this cohort basis for aggregation with the period basis. The cohort approach represents a longitudinal view; the period approach represents a cross-sectional view. We can illustrate this by reference again to the population pyramid in Figure 2-1.

Suppose that, in the census of January 1, 1900, each woman was asked to report any live births she had given during the calendar year 1900, the twelve months before the census. Aggregating on a period basis, we would represent all cohorts in the denominator and in the numerator only those births which occurred in the referent year, 1899. The simplest conventional measure of period fertility is the familiar *crude birth rate*, which includes in the denominator all survivors of all cohorts, regardless of sex or age.[e] The importance of the crude birth rate is its relation to the growth rate of the population.

The Necessity for Translation

In our attempt to trace back from fertility to marital events we are immediately faced with a paradox. We are used to thinking in period terms about fertility when we are relating fertility to population-growth problems; on the other hand, we are used to thinking in

---

[d]Conventionally, women aged fifty, or even forty-five, are presumed to have completed their periods of fecundity. Thus summaries of their fertility are presumed to refer to completed cohort fertility. Measures of fertility to cohorts of younger age have to be interpreted in view of the possible childbearing years remaining, but we will not encounter that problem in this book.

[e]Another conventional measure of period fertility is the general fertility rate which also is a cross section of cohorts, but which includes in the denominator only that part of the cross section relatively directly involved in the production of the children in the specified year: the women aged 15-49 (or 15-44) in the middle of the year.

cohort terms when we are relating fertility to marriage. Therefore, we have to translate from one frame of reference to the other at some stage of our path back along the causal chain. Let us elaborate this point.

The population characteristic cited as the core of most population problems is the annual growth rate of the population, present and projected. Annual population growth rates are period rates. Assuming negligible net migration, the annual growth rate of a population is equal to the annual (period) crude birth rate minus the annual (period) crude death rate. So when laymen talk of zero population growth, they generally are talking about annual (period) crude birth rates balancing annual (period) crude death rates.

On the other hand, when demographers study the impact of marital patterns upon fertility, they seem automatically to shift to the cohort frame of reference. The Davis-Blake list of intermediate variables between cultural patterns and fertility is easier to employ in cohort terms than in period terms, as we shall see in the next chapter. Attempts made to estimate the potential impact of delayed average age at marriage generally are couched in cohort terms.[1]

Since translation from the period approach to the cohort approach evidently will be necessary at some stage in our planned inquiry, we choose to make the conceptual translation now.[2] Two aspects of female cohort fertility impinge upon period fertility in the long run: (1) cohort completed fertility and (2) cohort age at childbearing. Let us treat them in that order.

Period Fertility and Cohort Completed Fertility

By cohort completed fertility we mean the average number of live births ever had by the survivors of a birth cohort of women by the time they completed their years of biological fecundity, say by age fifty. The relationship between cohort completed fertility and period fertility is simply stated: the lower the average completed fertility of cohorts, the lower the period fertility of population including those cohorts during the time that those cohorts are in their childbearing years.

Laymen are used to this relationship. So when advocates of zero (period) population growth say that such a zero growth implies a little more than two offspring per woman (in cohort terms), assuming low mortality and negligible migration, most people are able to follow the reasoning.

Of course, other factors can confound the tendency for lower cohort completed fertility to result in lower period fertility. Prominent among these is temporary imbalance in the relative size of female cohorts.

A dramatic contemporary illustration is the large size of the U.S. female birth cohorts of, say, the years from 1946 through 1957 due to the postwar "baby boom." The swollen size of these cohorts will tend to push period fertility upward during those years, already upon us, when members of these cohorts are in their childbearing ages. That this has not resulted in an appreciable rise in period fertility can be attributed to a *balancing downward force*, a change downward in the childbearing patterns of the cohorts involved: Females of the U.S. baby-boom cohorts reportedly are acting in a way which will bring them lower cohort completed fertility than their mothers.[3]

Period Fertility and Cohort
Age at Childbearing

If we knew the age of the mother at each childbirth experienced by the cohort before the exhaustion of fecundity, say age fifty, and computed some average of those ages, the result would be the average female age at childbearing for the cohort. It refers to the timing of the births, as distinguished from the total births finally produced. There are three paths by which delaying this timing could reduce period fertility without reducing the cohort completed fertility. All of these were elaborated a decade ago by Ansley J. Coale and C.Y. Tye.[4]

1. *Spreading Cohort Births Over a Larger Number of Years.* We can illustrate this by contrasting a pair of hypothetical situations represented by two countries, A and B. Suppose in both countries the cohort completed fertility is precisely the same, a completed family of two boys and two girls. Suppose, however, that in the case of country A the average age of the mothers at the time of birth of their daughters was twenty-five years and that in the case of country B the

average age of mothers at the time of birth of their daughters was thirty-five years. Should this situation persist, then daughters born in 1970 in country A would produce their daughters around 1995 while the daughters born in 1970 in country B would have to wait to around 2005 to do the same. And this would happen in every succeeding cohort of women. The result would be that the same number of births would be allocated to fewer years in country A than in country B. Thus on a per-year (period) basis, fertility would be higher in country A than in country B while on a cohort basis fertility would remain the same.

2. *Reducing the Proportion of Cohort Members Who Survive through Childbearing.* To illustrate this path, let us take the same hypothetical situation used above: country A in which the average age of mothers at the birth of their daughters was twenty-five years and country B where the average age was thirty-five years. Let us now bring in the factor of mortality. In both countries mortality will gradually deplete the members of each cohort from the moment of their simultaneous birth until the last member has died. Let us assume, further, that the schedule of mortality—the rate at which cohorts are depleted—is stable and the same for country A and country B.

Fewer members of the birth cohorts in country B will live through all their childbearing years than in country A. Thus the number of births per original member of the birth cohort in country B will be less than per original member of the birth cohort in country A.[f]

To reiterate, via the first path, whatever children are produced by female birth cohorts are spread over a larger number of years, thus reducing the annual (period) birth rates. Via the second path, the proportions of female birth cohorts surviving to produce all their scheduled children are reduced.

The two effects described so far are independent of each other. But they are cumulative in the sense that a delay in the age of childbearing would result in a decrease in period fertility by both avenues under normal conditions.

---

[f]As Coale and Tye have pointed out, the degree of fertility reduction coming from delay in childbearing via this path depends upon the growth rate of the population. Populations with high growth rates, and high birth rates, are the very ones in which a reduction in fertility via this path would be the most marked. Indeed, it even might operate in the opposite direction if there were a sizable negative population growth rate. See Coale and Tye, reference note 4, p. 637.

Finally, both of these paths of effect are potentially permanent. That is, a persistent difference in average age of childbearing would result in a persistent difference in period fertility by these paths, all else being equal. On the other hand, the third path of effect is transitional and would have an influence only while the average age of childbearing was in the process of changing.

3. *Depleting the Number of Births during the Period of Transition.* Suppose, in our country X, there had been a pattern of childbearing such that all women produced four children when the women were between ages twenty and thirty and then stopped childbearing forever. Suppose, by some decree, in 1900, women were suddenly forbidden from bearing any children before age thirty, but that the women later proceeded to produce their four children each between the ages of thirty and forty. There would be no births between 1900 and 1910; period fertility would be zero for those years. And these lost babies would be replaced only if, for some reason, twenty-year-olds were again allowed to bear children according to the former pattern.

How much is the potential negative effect of delay in childbearing by these three paths combined? Coale and Tye attempted to demonstrate this in a case which would be possible in underdeveloped countries. They took the fertility of India in 1956, held cohort completed fertility constant, but moved the age of childbearing gradually later over a ten-year period so that at the end the mean length of generation was 2.7 years later than it had been before the transition.[5] The long-run period fertility declined about 8 percent. In the shorter run, during the decade when the transition was taking place, the period fertility was temporarily reduced considerably below even that.

Summary

Fertility can be viewed either longitudinally, as the performance of a cohort of women through their lifetimes, or cross-sectionally, as the performance of a series of cohorts during a given short period of time such as a year. In the context of population growth problems, fertility usually is conceived in period terms rather than cohort terms; thus zero population growth means a balance between births and deaths in a given year.

Period fertility is determined by two distinct aspects of the fertility behavior of cohorts—the total births eventually produced by the cohort and the average age at which the women in the cohort produce those births. Increasing the age at childbearing of mothers in cohorts reduces period fertility by lengthening the time it takes newborn daughters to become mothers, by allowing more chance for mortality to deplete cohorts before they complete their childbearing, and by temporarily depleting the number of births during the period of transition from early childbearing to late childbearing.

It is important, in future chapters, to seek the determinants both of cohort completed fertility and of cohort female age at child-bearing.

3 Cohort Fertility and Marital Status

With this chapter we take as our dependent variable cohort fertility rather than period fertility. Our task is to continue to trace back from cohort completed fertility and cohort age at childbearing along the causal chain toward marital events, describing the nature of the links as we go. In the first section of the chapter, I develop a conceptual framework to assist us.

Modification of the Davis-Blake Framework

In this task I start with the familiar and classic Davis-Blake analytical framework specifying the variables intermediate between culture and fertility.[1] The scheme is presented unabbreviated as Figure 3-1, below.

The major classes (I, II, and III) were distinguished on the basis of their time relation in the reproductive process.

The process of reproduction involves three necessary steps sufficiently obvious to be generally recognized in human culture: (1) intercourse, (2) conception, and (3) gestation and parturition. In analyzing cultural influences on fertility, one may well start with the factors directly connected with these three steps. Such factors would be those through which, and only through which, cultural conditions *can* affect fertility. For this reason, by way of convenience, they can be called the "intermediate variables." . . . [2]

The marital patterns whose influence we want to understand fall clearly into Class IA, those factors "governing the formation and dissolution of (sexual) unions in the reproductive period." Figure 3-2 presents our modification of the Davis-Blake framework. The major changes are (a) the placement of the union variables (Davis-Blake Class IA) in a different relation to the other intermediate variables and (b) the confinement of sexual-union variables to marital unions alone. Let me explain.

Upon reflection, we can see that Davis-Blake Class IA belongs to a

```
I. Factors Affecting Exposure to Intercourse
   ("Intercourse Variables").
   A. Those governing the formation and dissolution of unions in the reproductive period.
      1. Age of entry into sexual unions.
      2. Permanent celibacy: proportion of women never entering sexual unions.
      3. Amount of reproductive period spent after or between unions.
         a. When unions were broken by divorce, separation, or desertion.
         b. When unions were broken by death of husband.
   B. Those governing the exposure to intercourse within unions.
      4. Voluntary abstinence.
      5. Involuntary abstinence (from impotence, illness, unavoidable but temporary separations).
      6. Coital frequency (excluding periods of abstinence).
II. Factors Affecting Exposure to Conception
    ("Conception Variables").
      7. Fecundity or infecundity, as affected by involuntary causes.
      8. Use or nonuse of contraception.
         a. By mechanical or chemical means.
         b. By other means.
      9. Fecundity or infecundity, as affected by voluntary causes (sterilization, subincision, medical
         treatment, etc.).
III. Factors Affecting Gestation and Successful Parturition
     ("Gestation Variables").
      10. Foetal mortality from involuntary causes.
      11. Foetal mortality from voluntary causes.
```

Figure 3-1. The Davis-Blake Classification of Intermediate Variables. Source: Davis and Blake, p. 212 (see note 1).

```
Marital-Union Variables: Those Governing the Formation and Dissolution of Marital Unions in the
Reproductive Period.
      1. Age of entry into marital unions.
      2. Permanent nonmarriage: proportion of women never entering marital unions.
      3. Amount of reproductive period spent after or between marital unions.
         a. When unions were broken by divorce or separation.
         b. When unions were broken by death of spouse.
```

```
Intercourse Variables: Those Governing the Exposure to Intercourse.
      4. Voluntary abstinence.
      5. Involuntary abstinence (from impotence, illness, unavoidable but temporary separations).
      6. Coital frequency (excluding period of abstinence).
Conception Variables: Factors Affecting Exposure to Conception.
      7. Fecundity or infecundity as affected by involuntary causes.
      8. Use or nonuse of contraception.
      9. Fecundity or infecundity as affected by voluntary causes (sterilization, etc.).
Gestation Variables: Factors Affecting Gestation and Successful Parturition.
      10. Foetal mortality from involuntary causes.
      11. Foetal mortality from voluntary causes.
```

```
Cohort Fertility: Completed Fertility and Age at Childbearing.
```

Figure 3-2. Modification of the Davis-Blake Classification.

logical set different from Classes IB, II, and III in one important respect: Class IA variables cannot influence fertility *directly*. Variable Class IB (exposure to intercourse within unions) can influence fertility directly, not necessarily by means of influencing other variable classes such as conception variables (Class II) or gestation variables (Class III). Similarly, the conception variables (Class II) can have a direct influence on fertility, not necessarily an indirect one by means of gestation variables (Class III). Thus all major classes of variables can bear directly on fertility except one—Class IA, the factors influencing the formation and dissolution of unions. Being in a sexual union influences fertility only to the degree that being in such a union influences exposure to intercourse, the likelihood of conception with intercourse, or the likelihood of successful gestation and parturition after conception. Thus in Figure 3-2 the Union Variables are seen as influencing the intercourse, conception, and gestation variables and thence cohort fertility.

The second major modification of the Davis-Blake framework is to discard the concept of "sexual union," referred to in their Class IA, in favor of "marital union." Let us define a *marital union* as a union in which coitus *and reproduction* are socially sanctioned.[a]

One reason for this change is the vagueness of the meaning of "sexual union." Clearly that concept was not intended to mean a single act of coitus, since then Class IA (those factors governing the formation and dissolution of unions) would be synonymous with Class IB (those factors governing the exposure to intercourse within unions). But there is considerable range between a single act of coitus and membership in a union in which coitus and reproduction are sanctioned, a marital union. What within that range was meant to be included within the concept of "sexual union" is not clear from Davis and Blake's article.

Another reason for the change is that the concept has not achieved currency since its introduction. Few, if any, other scholars have adopted the concept and integrated it into their conceptual frameworks. Indeed, whatever their original intentions, Davis and Blake themselves confine their attention largely to marital unions rather than other sexual unions in the later substantive part of the article in which they introduced the concept of sexual union.[3]

---

[a]In this we are following the Davis and Blake definition of marital union and also that of Hajnal. John Hajnal, "European Marriage Patterns in Perspective," in D.V. Glass and D.E.C. Eversley (eds.) *Population in History* (London: Arnold, 1965), pp. 104-105.

We seem, therefore, to be left with the choice of either reviving the concept of sexual unions and arbitrarily clarifying its meaning or continuing to treat it with the benign neglect it has enjoyed since its initial appearance. Let us choose the latter.

However, our substitution of the concept of marital unions for sexual unions does not free us of all conceptual difficulties. If marital unions are those in which coitus and reproduction are socially sanctioned, then who is the relevant sanctioning authority? Are we to treat the legal recognition of the marriage by the state as the criterion? Or are we to include unions in which reproduction is sanctioned by the community even though not by the legal system of the state? Strategic judgments on this score are difficult to make on any general basis without reference to the specific theoretical problem at hand. Thus we face this issue in the context of Chapter 4, "Fertility of the Nonmarried."

One additional change is necessary to accommodate the rest of the framework to our change from sexual unions to marital unions. Davis and Blake had the Intercourse Variables (IB) refer only to inter- course within sexual unions. In confining our attention to a subclass, marital unions, we raise the problem of how to deal with coitus outside of marital unions. Our answer is to have the intercourse variables refer to all intercourse, whether inside or outside of marital unions.

This has the advantage of allowing identification of illegitimate fertility as a separate class of outcome, something not possible with the original Davis-Blake framework. Thus a final reason for using "marital union" rather than "sexual union" is the resulting explicit treatment of illegitimacy permitted, such as in Chapter 4.

With the framework thus modified, we can state our guiding question for the present chapter more clearly: How does membership in a union in which coitus and reproduction are socially sanctioned influence behavior with respect to intercourse, conception, and gestation and thus influence cohort completed fertility and age at childbearing?[b,c]

---

[b]This is not meant to imply that marital union variables are the only ones influencing the intercourse, conception, and gestation variables and thus cohort fertility. In several places, Ronald Freedman has presented a classification of the independent variables which influence the Davis-Blake intermediate variables and thus fertility. That classification is summarized in an earlier article, David Yaukey, "On Theorizing about Fertility," *The American Sociologist* 4 (May 1969): 101.

[c]An alternative approach to ordering the relationship between age at marriage and fertility is presented in Joan Busfield, "Age at Marriage and Family Size: Social Causation and Social Selection Hypotheses," *Journal of Biosocial Science* 4 (1972): 117-134.

Female Cohort Marital Status

Since our dependent variable, fertility, is stated in cohort terms, we should conceive of our marital-union variables in cohort terms as well.

A cohort of women start out in *single* status. As they approach maturity, a majority of them will marry and thus take on the status of *married*. With time, some of the married women have *divorces* or their husbands die and *widow* them, thus putting them back into the status of *nonmarried,* along with their single contemporaries. Finally, some of these women who had been married but who had their marriages dissolved, will *remarry*, and again will take on the status of *married*, along with their contemporaries who never had their first marital unions dissolve.[d]

It is important to separate out two aspects of this cohort history for analytical purposes: marital *events* and marital *status*. It is by the occurrence of marital events (marriage, death of husband, voluntary marital dissolution, remarriage) that one changes one's marital status.

To me it seems primarily marital status, and not marital events, that bears directly on the Davis-Blake intermediate variables and thus on cohort fertility. Specifically, it is the distinction between the status of currently married and nonmarried that is of primary importance. To the degree that marital-union variables influence fertility, it is primarily because people in the status of married behave differently than they would have had they been nonmarried with respect to intercourse, conception, or gestation variables.[e] This view of the relation between marital events, marital status, and fertility is summarized in Figure 3-3.

The relationship between marital events and marital status in cohort histories is treated in Chapters 5 and 6. The complex manner in which the combined forces of marriage, male mortality, and voluntary marital dissolution influence married-nonmarried composi-

---

[d]All during this history, female mortality will have been depleting the birth cohort, so in fact we are describing the history of the survivors of the cohort at any given time after the date of cohort birth.

[e]I am inhibited from making a flat claim that marital events have no influence on fertility behavior other than through marital status by a lingering uncertainty that there might be some weak direct connections. For instance, let us suppose that a given couple first married in January 1960 and stayed married during that calendar year. Let us suppose, for contrast, that the same couple had become married in January 1959 and had stayed married all through calendar years 1959 and 1960. Should we assume that their behavior with respect to the intermediate variables during 1960 was not influenced by the timing of events? They were in the status of married during 1960 in each case.

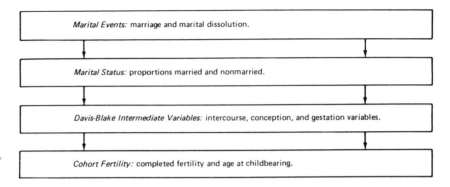

Figure 3-3. Relation between Marital Events and Fertility.

tion of the female cohort over time is too complex for brief treatment here. Our immediate task is to describe cohort marital status as a variable.

We can think of a female cohort's fertility history as having three major stages: the prefecund stage ending at age fifteen, the fecund stage extending from age fifteen through forty-nine, and the post-fecund stage extending from age fifty on.[f] The proportion of women married in the prefecund and postfecund stages are of no importance to us since being married could not influence their fertility in any case. Fertility is negligible whether they are married or not.

It behooves us to divide these remaining 35 "fecund" years between 15 and 49 into a series of substages in order to study the relation between marital status and fertility at each stage separately. The main reason for this precaution is that fecundity varies immensely in degree with age within the supposedly fecund years.[g] Moreover, the interrelationships between marital status and the other intermediate variables might well vary from one age stage to the next. Demographers conventionally divide the fertile years into five-year classes: 15-19, 20-24, 25-29, 30-34, 35-39, 40-44, and 45-49.[h]

---

[f]Demographers split as to whether 44 or 49 should be used as the final year of the female fecund years.

[g]For a more complete treatment of the age pattern of fecundity and related variables, see the section "Contingent Conditions: Female Age" in this chapter.

[h]The United Nations has observed that the pattern of relative fertility of the five-year female age periods from age 15 through 44 appears rather standard, whether the country has generally high fertility or generally low fertility. On the basis of this, the United Nations has

Following that convention, an ideal description of a cohort's marital status would consist of a series of seven proportions (percents). The denominator of each proportion would be the total woman-years lived by the survivors of the cohort during the specified five years of age: the total years of exposure to fertility. The numerator would be the number of those woman-years which were spent in the status of married.[i]

World Variation in Marital Status

Marital status can be a determinant of fertility differences among countries only if marital status composition varies among countries. Demonstrating the degree of international marital status variation in cohort terms is complicated by the practice of nations reporting marital status in cross-sectional terms. That is, a nation will take a census on a given date and present the marital statuses reported by all women on that date, by women's age on the census date, even though the reporting women belong not to one cohort but a series of them

Cross-sectional marital status distributions differ from cohort marital status histories when there have been changes in marital patterns during the histories of the cohorts being represented in the cross section. Nevertheless, world variations in cross-sectional marital status are at least indicative of the major contrasts in cohort marital status composition in the world. This is true because the major contrasts among cross-sectional types are so large that changes within the lifetime of cohorts represented are not likely to obscure them completely.

Using census data almost entirely from post-World War II, Bourgeois-Pichat has isolated five patterns of marital status composition by female age.[4] These are presented as Figure 3-4. The five types

---

used a set of weights to represent the relative fertility of age classes from 15-19 through 40-44: 1, 7, 7, 6, 4, 1. United Nations, *Manual III: Methods of Population Projections by Sex and Age.* (New York: United Nations, 1956), pp. 42-44.

[i]The concept of cohort marital status is related to, but not synonymous with, that of the family cycle, introduced by Paul C. Glick and his associates. A description of the family cycle consists of stating the average ages at which specified events occur in the life of a cohort. Glick's early work used cross-sectional data to construct synthetic cohorts, but his more recent work has employed actual cohort data. Paul C. Glick and Robert Parke, "New Approaches in the Studying of the Life Cycle of the Family," *Demography* (1965): 187-202. Also see Andrew Collver, "The Family Cycle in India and the United States," *American Sociological Review* 28 (February 1963): 86-96.

Femmes mariées suivant l'âge (pour 100)

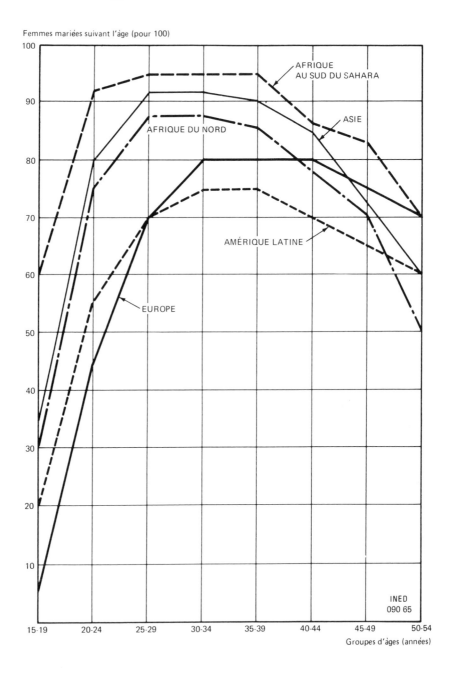

Figure 3-4. Five Contemporary Types of Marital Status Composition. Source: Bourgeois-Pichat, graphique no. 1, p. 389 (see note 4).

are Africa south of the Sahara, North Africa, Asia, Latin America, and Europe (including Australia, New Zealand, and the United States).[j]

Bourgeois-Pichat dramatizes the difference among these types by a summary estimation of the proportion of the potentially fertile years spent in a married state for each type. He sets the figure 100 to represent the hypothetical situation in which all women are married from age fifteen through fifty-four and no woman dies in the interim. He then computes a figure for each of the five types representing what percentage of that time would be spent in the married state for the type, again assuming no women died in the period. The index figures are 84.8 for Africa south of the Sahara, 75.7 for Asia, 69.5 for North Africa, 62.5 for Europe, and 61.2 for Latin America.[k]

Contingent Conditions: Female Age

If our conceptual framework is valid, then cohort marital status can influence period fertility only by influencing one or more of the Davis-Blake intercourse, conception, or gestation variables. That is, a high proportion nonmarried in a cohort of females reduces the cohort fertility only because nonmarried women behave differently from married women with respect to intercourse variables (either abstaining for long periods or having a lower general frequency), with respect to conception variables (having lower fecundability or using contraception more effectively), or with respect to gestation variables (having more stillbirths and abortions, spontaneous or induced). Such differences in behavior with respect to the intermediate variables can influence period fertility either by reducing the average completed fertility of the cohort or by delaying the average age of mothers at the birth of their children for the cohort.

---

[j]The variation among types would be even greater if the chart included the pre-World War II "European pattern" of late marriage and large proportions never marrying identified by Hajnal.[5]

[k]Bourgeois-Pichat, "Facteurs de la Fecondite," p. 390. This method can be seen as a translation of cross-sectional observations into cohort terms by using the concept of synthetic cohorts. One supposes that a hypothetical cohort actually experienced a marital-status composition history identical to the one found by cross-sectional observations from a census. In fact this supposition is unlikely, but the technique allows concise summary measures.

The differences between married and nonmarried fertility behavior are not always complete. We shall deal with fertility of the nonmarried in Chapter 4. However, for the sake of orderly presentation, let us assume for the moment that societies are in fact successful in eliminating all fertility other than marital fertility. The question we should now approach is: Under what conditions would a reduction of the proportion of cohort women who were married result in a maximum proportional reduction of fertility?

A contingent condition of major importance is female age. Fecundity varies with female age during the years 15-49. Therefore, it makes considerable difference from which age period time is being lost through nonmarriage. Nonmarriage would have maximal negative effect on completed cohort fertility if the cohort years in nonmarried status tended to fall in the most fecund age periods.

Empirically, the usual case is quite the opposite. Let us take the age pattern of maximal uncontrolled fertility and chart a curve for it in Figure 3-5. These values, estimated by Ansley Coale, represent "the highest fertility any whole nation might be expected to attain" in the absence of birth control.[6] We also have included in the same figure one of Bourgeois-Pichat's marital-status by age types, the one for Asia, taken from our Figure 3-4. One can see that generally, the ages with the greatest proportion nonmarried are those with the lowest uncontrolled fertility. In short, the age pattern of nonmarriage in regions such as Asia severely limit the loss of fertility through nonmarriage.[l]

The factors contributing to such an age pattern of uncontrolled fertility as in Figure 3-5 could be complex. One factor could be the rise and fall of female fecundability, the probability of conception in a given menstrual cycle for a woman exposed to intercourse.[m] Another could be a change in frequency of coitus with age. Yet another could be change in ability to carry conceptions safely to term.

We have a relatively clear understanding of the factors involved

---

[l]From a functional viewpoint it seems plausible that societies protecting high fertility to balance historical high mortality would have norms maximizing the proportions of female fecund years spent in unions where reproduction was sanctioned.

[m]United Nations, Department of Economic and Social Affairs, *Multilingual Demographic Dictionary-English Section,* (New York: United Nations, 1958), p. 41. "Fecundity" is a more inclusive concept, defined as "the capacity of a man, a woman or a couple to participate in reproduction." Ibid., p. 38.

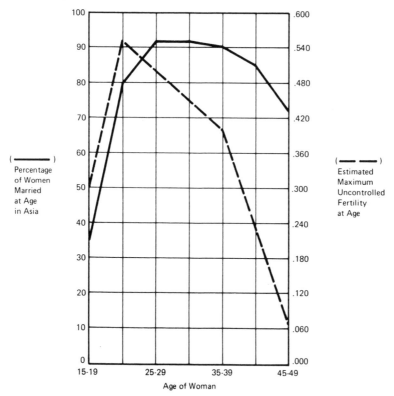

Figure 3-5. Age Patterns of Uncontrolled Fertility and Married Status. Sources: Bourgeois-Pichat, table IC (see note 4); and Coale, table 1 (see note 6).

with regard to increase in uncontrolled fertility from the teens to the early twenties. It is dominantly due to the increase in fecundability, the likelihood of conception with intercourse.[7] This hypothesis is confirmed, for instance, by the longer delays between marriage and first conception for noncontracepting teenage brides as contrasted to brides marrying in their twenties.[8]

The reasons for the later decline in uncontrolled fertility, say from age thirty to fifty, is less clear. Henry expresses developing skepticism that the main factor is a decline in fecundability. Rather he points to the increasing evidence of marked increases in risk of fetal mortality with age of mother.[9] To this one should add any effect of a decline in frequency of coitus and any decline in the male sperm count per coitus, indirect factors brought into play by the tendency for older women to have older partners.

Whatever the causes of the curve of uncontrolled fertility shown in Figure 3-5, we can use it for some guidance in answering our question: Under what conditions would a reduction of the proportion of a cohort who were married result in a maximal proportional reduction of fertility? To reduce the average cohort *completed fertility* to the greatest degree, one should concentrate on reducing the proportion married during the twenties, and especially in the early twenties. Reduction of the proportion married in the teens, and especially the early teens, will not have the same impact on cohort completed fertility. Indeed, that is the basis of much of the debate as to the importance or effect of delaying age at first marriage in India, where most of the delay from present averages would result in loss of woman-years in the teens.[n]

At a given level of cohort completed fertility, *age at childbearing* would be increased by minimizing the fertility of young women in contrast with older women. In order to maximize age at childbearing by changing cohort marital status, one would focus on those ages which produce most children with young mothers, the years where women are both youngest and most fecund. Thus this factor focuses our attention even more on the earlier ages of the fecund years: the twenties and especially the early twenties. In addition, it cautions us against dismissing the teens as having no potential influence. Even though fecundity is relatively low then, those children that are produced in women's teens have a maximal effect on shortening the length of generations.

---

[n]However, an indirect effect of early childbearing might be damaging of the female reproductive apparatus which would reduce a woman's fecundity throughout the rest of her normally fecund years, thus lowering her completed fertility. For estimates of the effect of delay in age of women at first marriage on cohort completed fertility in India, see Maurari Majumdar and Ajit Das Gupta, "Marriage Trends and Their Demographic Implications," *Sankyha*, ser. B 31 (3-4); Calcutta (December 1969), pp. 491-500; S.N. Agarwala, "The Effect of a Rise in Female Marriage Age on Birth Rate in India," in United Nations Department of Economic and Social Affairs, *Proceedings of the World Population Conference 1965* (New York: United Nations, 1967), p. 172; N.C. Das, "A Note on the Effect of Postponement of Marriage on Fertility," in United Nations Department of Economic and Social Affairs, *Proceedings of the World Population Conference 1965*, pp. 128-30;

Contingent Conditions:
Fecundity Selectivity

Fecundity differences, however, are not entirely due to female age. Women of the same age vary considerably in their fecundity. If so, we should try to specify under what condition, regarding distribution of fecundity at given female ages, a given reduction in the proportion married would result in a maximum reduction in cohort completed fertility. The condition would be having the most fecund women in the married status before the supposed reduction in the proportion married. If the subfecund women had also been the married women, then relatively little fertility would be lost by taking them out of the married status.

Whether that condition is normally met is a matter of conjecture and probably also of considerable international variation. For selection on the basis of fecundity can occur at the stage of first marriage, of marital dissolution, and of remarriage. Here are some plausible but tentative examples to illustrate the possibilities.

High fecundity might hasten first marriage. Under a given set of conditions regarding coital frequency and contraceptive efficiency, the more fecundable women are by definition the most likely to conceive. Thus, other things being equal, they also would be the more likely to marry early in order to legitimate their children. Presumably this avenue would be most operative where there is widespread premarital pregnancy but not widespread illegitimacy or induced abortion. For instance, Bumpass found indirect evidence of young marriage being selective with respect to fecundity in the United States.[10] The result would be that, in the earliest age categories, the married women would tend to be relatively fecund compared with the nonmarried women.

Moreover, less fecund women may be more likely to suffer marital dissolution. For instance, a major reason for divorce in Moslem societies is supposed to be the infertility of the woman. It also is possible that women who are more likely to have difficulty in gestation and parturition also are more likely to die in childbirth.

Another avenue by which the most fecund women might be selected for marriage is by selective remarriage. Men seeking fecund wives can make fecundity inferences about candidates on the basis of marital performance during women's previous marriages. If further fertility is desired, men may marry the apparently more fecund women. On the other hand, if men choose not to have additional children, or if they choose not to adopt many already living children of the women, they might actually select subfecund women for remarriage. For example, Driver presents evidence from India that widows of lower past fertility had better chances of remarriage.[11]

It probably is true that by these combined avenues the fecundity of the married vs. nonmarried female population, at given ages, is biased. But the direction of the influence and the net degree of influence in one direction or the other is far too complex to conjecture as a generality.

Contingent Conditions:
Birth Control

Probably the most important contingent condition affecting the relationship between marital status and period fertility is the degree of voluntary control over fertility exercised, whether it be through contraception or induced abortion. To illustrate, let us assume that all women in the cohort want to have exactly three live births. Let us assume further that the women are completely effective in avoiding unwanted births while having sexual contact with husbands. Finally, let us assume that the women choose to have these three children in rapid succession, over a five-year period. If the cohort all marries at age twenty, then each woman will have the three children between ages twenty and twenty-five; if the cohort all marries at age twenty-five, then each will have the three children between ages twenty-six and thirty. Under this kind of condition, the influence of a change in marital status on *completed fertility* of the survivors of the cohort has been *nil*.

The conditions under which women voluntarily could nullify the effect of marital status composition on cohort completed fertility would be (1) where the desired family size was small enough not to require all of the fecund years to reach the desired size, (2) where cohort marital histories were such that the woman-years of nonmarriage were spread among all the women rather than some women having histories with no married years at all. Under such extreme conditions, it is conceivable that a reduction of the proportion married by, say, 20 percent at all ages would have no influence on average completed fertility for women in the cohort.

Nevertheless, the voluntary compensating behavior women would be engaging in still would influence period fertility by means of delaying average *age at childbearing*. That is, women who were nonmarried at earlier ages would be making up for their early infertility by having their desired children at later ages. Therefore, a greater proportion of the women in the cohort would die before completing the average fertility that would be experienced by surviving members of the cohort. And the average length of generations would be increased, thus spreading the cohort births over a larger number of years.[o]

Thus the introduction of effective voluntary control over fertility, under the conditions of limited desired family size, would have a complex effect on period fertility. Although voluntary control might reduce the effect of nonmarriage on cohort completed fertility, by the same process it would tend to increase the age of women at childbearing. Voluntary control over fertility might dampen the effect of increased nonmarriage on cohort fertility, but it would not eliminate it.

Summary

The task of this chapter was to develop a conceptual framework for tracing the relationships between marital patterns and cohort fertility. We employed as a starting point the exhaustive Davis-Blake taxonomy of variables intermediate between cultural factors and fertility. We found it convenient to modify the Davis-Blake framework in two important respects: First, we restricted their class of variables affecting the formation and dissolution of sexual unions so it referred only to marital unions, defined as unions in which coitus and reproduction were socially sanctioned. Second, we cast marital-union variables not in the role of variables intermediate between culture and fertility but rather as part of the cultural patterns which influence the remaining Davis-Blake variables and thus influence fertility.

---

[o]For a more complete specification of how age at childbearing influences period fertility, see Chapter 2.

A further step in developing the conceptual framework was that of articulating the marital-union variables as they applied to the history of actual cohorts. A distinction was made between marital statuses and the marital events, which marked the change from one marital status to another. In our framework, marital status is seen to have direct effect on fertility-determining behavior and marital events to influence primarily through determining marital status histories of cohorts.

Having identified cohort marital status as an independent variable of import, we touched on problems of description. It was judged most important to register the proportion of women-years lived by the cohort which were in the married status, registered separately for five-year age classes ranging from fifteen through about forty-nine. To illustrate the international variety that might be expected in cohort marital status histories, we cited the international typology by Bourgeois-Pichat.

The degree of the influence of marital status upon fertility can be seen to rest on contingent conditions, some of which we identified. The effect of nonmarried status on fertility is influenced, for instance, by the level of fecundity. Because of the age variation in fecundity, an increase in the proportion in the nonmarried status was seen as having the maximal negative impact on cohort fertility if it referred to the early twenties. However, since women vary in fecundity at the same age, either subfecund or superfecund women might be married at a given age, depending on a variety of possible cultural patterns of selectivity at the stage of first marriage, marital dissolution, or remarriage.

Another contingent condition affecting the relationship between marital union variables and cohort fertility is the degree of voluntary birth control in the society. Under extreme conditions of absolute effective control, low desired family size, and participation in adequate marital periods by all women wanting children, it is conceivable that reduction in proportions married would have no effect on cohort completed fertility. However, even under those circumstances it is likely that age at childbearing would be delayed and that period fertility would be reduced somewhat by that route.

This chapter's presentation assumed, for simplicity, that there was no reproduction outside of marital unions. That is a crucial simplification, since it is debatable whether the proportions nonmarried could be much changed without incurring a strain upon those methods of social control which have held fertility largely within marriage. For some insight into the likelihood of this assumption, in the following chapter we treat fertility of the nonmarried.

4

Fertility of the Nonmarried

This chapter is a tangent from the main line of the book. The main line leads from marital events to period fertility. Following that line, it is easy to forget that nonmarriage is not synonymous with nonfertility. The purpose of this chapter is to point out the consequences of ignoring illegitimate fertility.

We start by stating the normal assumptions regarding both (a) the degree of illegitimacy that is likely under conditions of late female age at marriage and (b) the means by which unmarried females are presumed to eliminate their fertility.[a] Evaluating those assumptions, it turns out, involves conceptual problems which we treat briefly. We then use recently-gathered evidence concerning Europe from about 1850 to 1940 to estimate the validity of the stated assumptions with respect to that period. From that review, and on the basis of logical deduction, we hypothesize conditions under which delayed female age at marriage is most likely to result in high illegitimacy. The hypotheses lead us to unusual conclusions about the relationship between family-planning policies and delayed-marriage policies.

Two Common Assumptions

Some demographers have made explicit estimates of the effect on fertility of increasing the age of women at first marriage. Others have implied such estimates in their advocacy of policies to delay marriage in order to limit population growth. Any estimate of the fertility effect of delaying marriage employs assumptions about the fertility of unmarried women, whether the assumptions be stated or not.

One assumption, apparently universal, is that nonmarital fertility

---

[a]Age at first marriage is only one of the marital norms influencing cohort marital status and thus fertility. However, as Chapters 5 and 6 will detail, it is a dominant one in determining the proportion of *young* women who are nonmarried. Moreover, the policies of marital change yet proposed for fertility reasons have dealt almost exclusively with female age at first marriage. Thus, to simplify this chapter, we will deal only with one determinant of cohort marital status: age of woman at first marriage.

will remain negligible even with the supposed delay in marriage. In most formal estimates, this assumption is recognized, stated, and sometimes defended.[1] In statements advocating policies to delay marriage, the assumption normally is stated as a condition for the desired effect. Thus Kingsley Davis says that one way in which an improved population-control policy can reduce fertility is "by *keeping present controls over illegitimate childbirth* yet making the most of factors that lead people to postpone or avoid marriage."[2] (Italics added.)

A second assumption, usually implied, is that nonmarriage will influence fertility by means of limiting sexual intercourse, rather than, for instance, by increasing voluntary contraception or abortion. Delay of marriage is advocated particularly in those societies where voluntary birth control is not well established, presumably because it is seen as not requiring birth control as a means for influence on fertility.[3] More explicitly, Ryder states,

The modus operandi of fertility reduction must take one of three forms; reduction of the probability of intercourse; reduction of the probability of conception if intercourse occurs; reduction of the probability of birth if conception occurs. *The first of these control through nuptiality* ... the latter two constitute control of marital fertility.[4] (Italics added.)

We suspect that the tendency to make this assumption is reinforced by an uncritical use of the original Davis-Blake analytical framework. Davis and Blake include "[factors] governing the formation and dissolution of unions" as a *subclass, contained within* the larger class of "factors affecting exposure to intercourse."[5]

In this second assumption, advocates of delayed marriage are following in the venerable footsteps of Thomas Malthus. He advocated "moral restraint" (the postponement of marriage with no extramarital sexual gratification) in contrast with "vice" (including birth control) as a preventive check against population growth. However, this advocacy of delayed marriage does not necessarily imply much confidence on his part that marital delay would in fact be accompanied by premarital abstinence. As Petersen points out, the scientist and the moralist were mixed in Malthus:[6] his advocacy of delayed marriage combined with premarital continence might have been more of a normative statement than a serious prediction that they would occur together. Indeed, one can find passages in which

Malthus seems kindly tolerant of those who might stray from his advocated path into extramarital intercourse, much in the manner of a parson who is sadly aware of sin in his flock.

I should be most extremely sorry to say any thing which could be either directly or remotely be construed unfavorably to the cause of virtue: but I certainly cannot think that the vices which relate to sex are the only vices which are to be considered in a moral question; or that they are even the greatest and most degrading to the human character. . . . A large class of women, and many men, I have no doubt, pass a considerable part of their lives in moral restraint; but I believe there will be found very few who pass through the ordeal of squalid and hopeless poverty, or even long continued embarrassed circumstances, without a considerable moral degradation of character.[7]

Specifying the Questions

Evaluating the two identified assumptions requires answering the following questions of fact: (1) To what degree does being nonmarried fail to prevent fertility? and (2) To the degree that being nonmarried does prevent fertility, by what means does it do so?

Let us try to answer these questions about Western Europe during its modernization in the nineteenth and early twentieth centuries. Before we can bring evidence to bear, however, we have to face some conceptual and logical problems.

On the face of it, answering question number one seems straightforward: count the illegitimate births. But to use the number of illegitimate births as the measure of the failure of nonmarriage to prevent fertility is to accept the government's definition of marriage. In Chapter 2 we defined a marital union as one in which coitus and reproduction are sanctioned. Left open in that definition is the specification of the sanctioning authority. Accepting the national government as the sanctioning authority leads one to deal arbitrarily with two important classes of unions which could be considered marital from other viewpoints.

The first class is *consensual unions*. Let us define these as unions in which reproduction is not sanctioned by the government but is sanctioned by one or more significant segments of the society to which the partners belong, such as a community or sect. As our attempt at definition demonstrates, this is not a homogeneous class of unions. It is, however, numerically significant in some regions and times. It is generally agreed that consensual unions involve sizable minorities of adult women in contemporary Latin America.[8] Nor should it be assumed that they are insignificant historically elsewhere, including parts of Europe.[9]

The second class we can call *premarital unions*, defined as those in which coitus is sanctioned on the condition that the couple be married before the birth to it. A quotation from Knodel will help to specify what we mean.

There is a substantial body of ethnographic evidence which describes widespread customs during preceding centuries permitting pre-marital intercourse in much of northern and central Europe. These customs apparently stemmed from old patterns of nocturnal visitation which were common in some rural areas during mediaeval times and persisted into the eighteenth and nineteenth centuries. According to these customs an unmarried man was permitted to sleep with an unmarried woman, and, if both partners were potential spouses, to have sexual relations. However, the couple were held responsible for offspring and when pregnancy occurred marriage would follow.[10]

Petersen describes the identical pattern for the Netherlands and translates its Dutch name as "window wooing."[11] With regard to England, Wrigley finds evidence of a similar pattern existing in Colyton for centuries before our period of reference.[12] We follow Shorter, Knodel, and Van de Walle, however, in distinguishing between such "institutionalization of intimacy in courtship patterns" on the one hand and "shotgun marriages" on the other.[13]

Should births resulting from premarital unions be used as evidence of the failure of nonmarriage to prevent fertility? One can argue either side of the question.

One can take the view that those premarital unions resulting in bridal pregnancies were cases of illegitimate conception if not illegitimate birth. Since conception preceded marriage, this argument might say, and since nonmarriage did not result in abortion before birth, then nonmarriage did not prevent the birth.

On the other hand, one can suppose that couples did not enter into the implied obligations of premarital unions, as we define them, until they were willing to follow through on the obligation to marriage on a few months notice. If that be so, their ability, eligibility, and willingness to marry in the immediate future was a prerequisite to their entering premarital unions. From this viewpoint, couples in premarital unions were nonmarried only in a superficial sense; they already were in unions in which reproduction would be sanctioned as soon as it was imminent. Thus bridal pregnancies would not be evidence of the failure of nonmarriage to prevent fertility.[b]

However, probably not all bridal pregnancies resulted in premarital unions of the conditional sort supposed above. An unknown proportion did involve "shotgun marriages," where the partners had no intention of ultimate marriage to each other in the event of conception, but where they were nevertheless coerced into it after the woman conceived.[14]

No decision about how to treat bridal pregnancies seems entirely satisfactory. Therefore we are strongly swayed by technical considerations. Whereas illegitimate births are relatively accurately recorded, bridal pregnancies are not.

Let us include illegitimate births from consensual unions and exclude legitimate births resulting from bridal pregnancies as evidence of the failure of nonmarriage to prevent fertility. (Note that these inclusions and exclusions tend to counterbalance.) In other words, let us use all illegitimate births, as officially defined, as the measure of failure.

Our question number two is: To the degree that being nonmarried does prevent fertility, by what means does it do so? The problem is to find evidence with which to challenge the assumption that noncoitus is the sole means. Obviously it is difficult to find reliable records of extramarital coital frequency. Evidence of extramarital contraception of induced abortion would be presumptive evidence of extramarital coitus, but direct evidence again is lacking. Instead, we will have to rely on evidence of voluntary birth control *within* marriage. It seems more reasonable to suppose that prevention of extramarital fertility is being accomplished partially via birth control

---

[b]Bridal pregnancy also could have an impact on marital fertility, by two distinct paths: (1) It would increase the live births per woman during the first nine months of marriage; (2) it could present evidence for men to use in selecting women for marriage. With regard to the second path, (a) women of demonstrated subfecundity may be either sought or avoided as marital partners on that basis, but probably sought, and (b) highly fecund women, conceiving earlier under given conditions of coitus, would be more likely to marry early and thus spend more of their young years in marital unions. All of these influences on marital fertility probably would be positive, and especially so where large proportions of women marry late or never. See our presentation in Chapter 3, regarding the conditions under which cohort marital status influences fertility.

in a society where marital birth control is prevalent than in a society in which marital birth control is absent.

There are two reasons for selecting Europe during its modernization for initial study. The first is that Europe from 1800 or earlier to about 1940 was characterized by what Hajnal calls "the European pattern" of nuptiality, late average ages at first marriage and large proportions of women never marrying. Only under such unusual conditions of large proportions in the nonmarried state will we be able to find evidence about the concomitants of nonmarriage.[c]

The second reason is that relevant information has just been gathered and summarized in admirable detail. In 1964 a team headed by Ansley J. Coale started a study of the decline of fertility in Europe during the preceding century or so. In the process, the team paid special attention to marital patterns, and ultimately also to illegitimate fertility. Although the series of books which will finally report their work has just begun to appear, several preliminary articles are published.[15]

Europe 1850-1940:
Levels of Illegitimacy

The marriage pattern of most of Europe as it existed for at least two centuries up to 1940 was . . . unique or almost unique in the world. . . . The distinctive marks of the "European pattern" are (1) a high age at marriage and (2) a high proportion of women who never marry. . . . The European pattern extended over all of Europe to the west of a line running roughly from Leningrad to Trieste.[16]

Having said this, Hajnal proceeds to present evidence describing the "European pattern" of nuptiality. Since we are focusing on the

---

[c]Obviously the study of Europe 1850-1940 only begins an adequate investigation of the illegitimacy consequences of delayed marriage in a variety of cultural contexts. If we were to expand the effort on the historical level, we would pay particular attention to Ireland as a deviation from the general European case, 1850-1940. In more recent history, the rise in age at first marriage in Japan since World War II (and more recently in Korea, Hong Kong, Taiwan, Singapore, and Ceylon) furnishes another set of cultural circumstances. On a contemporary, cross-sectional basis, the study of Latin America should be extremely rewarding. In Latin American countries one finds variety in terms of normal age of women at first marriage (though most are late by world standards), in terms of prevalence of contraception, abortion, consensual unions, and illegitimacy, and in terms of technological development.

effects of female age at first marriage, we will pay especial attention to the proportion of women aged 20-24 who were single.[17] If we take 1900 as the year of reference, as does Hajnal, then Hajnal's figures show that proportion to run from 55 percent to 86 percent for the countries West of Hajnal's imaginary line and 44 percent or below for all European countries East of the line. Table 4-1 presents the data from Hajnal for countries West of the line.[18]

Turning from nonmarriage to illegitimate fertility, we present Figure 4-1, taken from one presented by Shorter, Knodel, and Van de Walle.[19] We will pay attention to time trends in the next section of the chapter. For the moment it is sufficient to notice that the peak levels of illegitimacy generally occurred around the period 1850 through 1880. Thus if one is interested in estimating the maximal failure of nonmarriage to prevent fertility, he should look to that period.

The index of illegitimacy is a measure developed by the Coale

Table 4-1
Percentage of Women Aged 20-24 Single in 1900

Country	Percentage Single
Ireland	86
Iceland	81
Sweden	80
Holland	79
Switzerland	78
Norway	77
Denmark	75
Great Britain	73
Germany	71
Belgium	71
Portugal	69
Finland	68
Austria	66
Italy	60
France	58
Spain[a]	55

[a]Age class 21-25 rather than 20-24.
Source: Hajnal, Table 2 (see note 16).

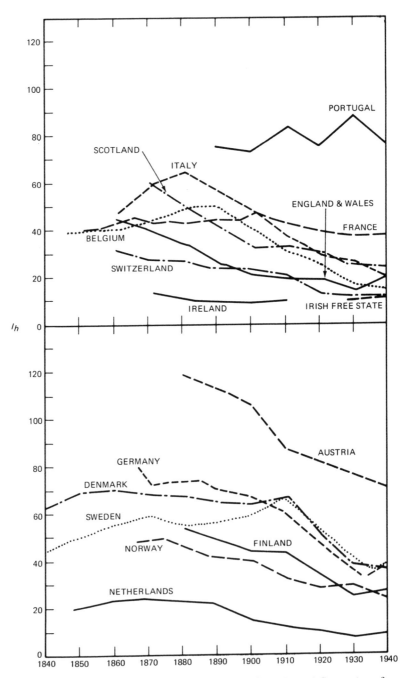

Figure 4-1. Index of Illegitimate Fertility (I_h), Selected Countries of Europe, 1840-1940. Source: Shorter, Knodel, and Van de Walle, figure I (see note 13).

team. The following quote from Shorter will acquaint the reader with its properties.

The index of illegitimate fertility is calculated as follows:

$$I_h = \frac{1,000\,B_I}{\sum u_i F_i}$$

where

B_I is the annual number of illegitimate births:

U_i is the number of nonmarried women in the ith age group between 15 and 49; and

F_i is the marital fertility of the Hutterites, the members of a religious sect of North Americans who do not practice contraception. . . .

The Index I_h is really just an illegitimate fertility rate (number of illegitimate births/1,000 unmarried women of childbearing age) which has been "indirectly" standardized for the age distribution of the unmarried women (this is important because of age differences in fertility). Finally the formula has been transformed by multiplying the number of women in each age bracket by the marital fertility of the Hutterite women in that age bracket. The Hutterites were selected as a reference population because they have the highest fertility on record. . . . An I_h of 40, for example, means that the unmarried women had 4% of the births expected from a group of married Hutterite women of the same age.[20]

Inspection of Figure 4-1 indicates that national I_h levels in 1850-1880 ranged from 120 for Austria to about 10 for Ireland, almost all of the remaining cases falling between 20 and 80. Thus, in almost all of the western European nations in 1850-80, the fertility of nonmarried women was between 2 and 8 percent of what married Hutterite women would have experienced at the same ages.

But *marital* fertility levels in Europe in the late 1880s were lower than the marital fertility rates of the Hutterites.[21] A more appropriate measure of the degree to which nonmarriage failed to prevent fertility would be a comparison between the age-specific illegitimate fertility and age-specific legitimate fertility rates for a given country. Unfortunately, summary figures for such a comparison are not available.[d] Our closest approximation is the *illegitimacy ratio*, which

[d]Van de Walle points out that one can multiply the I_h (index of illegitimate fertility) by the I_g (index of legitimate fertility) for a given country in order to take into account the degree to which marital fertility in that country is lower than Hutterite marital fertility. Private correspondence, November 20, 1972. Enabling tabular data were not presented in the Shorter, Knodel, Van de Walle article. However, visual comparisons can be made for the countries presented in our Figure 4-2, taken from Shorter, Knodel, and Van de Walle.

compares the total illegitimate births to the total legitimate births, without however controlling for the differences in the age compositions (and thus the fecundity compositions) of the populations of women.

Let us present what information we have been able to gather about illegitimacy ratios for the late 1800s. For Scandinavia, the earliest figures Kumar gives us are 1900 for Norway and Sweden; roughly 7 percent of all births in Norway and 12 percent in Sweden were illegitimate.[22] Livi-Bacci estimates that Portugal's level of illegitimacy was on a par with that of such northern European countries as Sweden, and higher than such Mediterranean countries as Italy and Spain.[23] He says that in 1858-62, 5.6 percent of all births were illegitimate in Spain.[24] For England and Wales, Hartley reports that 6.5 percent of births were illegitimate in 1851-60.[25]

Clearly fertility outside of marriage was a small fraction of what one would expect it to have been had these same women been married from the onset of fecundity. The reader, however, will make his own judgment as to the acceptability of the simplifying assumption that illegitimate fertility was negligible.[e]

Europe 1850-1940:
Time Patterns

Our intention is to review time patterns of illegitimacy, of nuptiality, and indirectly of fertility-determining behavior in western Europe from 1850-1940. The purpose is to suggest answers to our second

---

[e]As to the extent of bridal pregnancy in the area where premarital unions apparently were an accepted pattern, our best information is from England. Wrigley notes that in Colyton during the 1800s "about a third of all first children were baptised within eight months of marriage, many of these in the first three months." Wrigley, *Population and History*, p. 88. On the basis of parish registers for rural and semirural parishes in the early nineteenth century, Hair estimates that about two-fifths of all brides were pregnant. He also cites official statistics for 1938 to the effect that 18 percent of brides aged 15 to 45 in England and Wales were pregnant at marriage. P. Hair, "Bridal Pregnancy in Rural England in Earlier Centuries," *Population Studies* 20 (November 1966): 240. For the same area and the same year, Hartley provides evidence of the relative importance of bridal pregnancy compared with illegitimacy: of all the conceptions outside of marriage, about 70 percent were legitimated by marriage before the birth of the child. Hartley, "Rise of Illegitimacy," Table 3, p. 540.

question: To the degree that being nonmarried did prevent fertility, by what means did it do so?[f]

Let us start with a description of the status quo in 1850. According to Hajnal, the "European pattern" of nuptiality had been established for a century, more or less.[26] Illegitimacy levels were substantial compared with the traditional past.[27] Marital fertility rates were moderate, by worldwide standards, and generally stable.

The prevalence of voluntary birth control in Europe, prior to the general and continuous decline in fertility starting in the late 1800s, is unclear. A quotation from Ansley Coale expresses his uncertainty.

Our work to date has shown . . . that our initial framework of thought was oversimplified. The framework suggests that there should have been in every province during the pre-decline period of "natural fertility" a plateau of essentially constant I_g [marital fertility] . . . . But there are disturbing genuine indications that natural fertility is not as clear-cut a concept . . . as our preliminary framework of analysis suggests. . . . Indeed, there are a number of suggestions, direct or indirect, that the deliberate control of fertility in some form is latent in populations that have not begun a sustained and extended decline, opening up the possibility that there is a fraction, not changing in size, that for a long time practiced some form of deliberate fertility limitation.[28]

Let us turn to a description of the changes between the 1850s and World War II. With respect to nuptiality, there seem to be two national patterns during the period. One pattern is stability, exemplified by Sweden, England and Wales, Spain and Portugal.[29] The second pattern is a gradual and slight decrease in the average age at marriage and thus in the proportions nonmarried at early ages, this pattern showing in France, Switzerland, Belgium, the Netherlands, the German-speaking provinces of Austria-Hungary, and Germany.[30]

If the trends with respect to marriage are unclear, the trends with respect to illegitimacy are *not*.[31] To quote Shorter, Knodel, and Van de Walle, "Between 1880 and 1940, to take approximate dates, illegitimate fertility rates in Europe dropped precipitously, falling in most countries by 50 percent or more."[32] Our Figure 4-1, taken from Shorter, et al., demonstrates their point. In virtually every one

---

[f]The early limit of this period is defined by the absence of necessary systematic comparable official data for prior dates. The late limit is defined by the change in marital patterns, the "marriage boom" associated with World War II.

of the fifteen European countries presented, the index of illegitimate fertility (I_h) declined from 1880 through 1930.

Shorter, Knodel, and Van de Walle emphasize that the time trend in illegitimate fertility was closely associated with the time trend of the next factor we want to study: marital or legitimate fertility. The period 1880 to 1940 shows a precipitous decline in marital fertility throughout Europe. Shorter, et al., present us with evidence of this on a country by country basis in a chart abbreviated into Figure 4-2. For the ten countries presented, the pattern of change between 1880 and 1940 is generally downward in parallel for both the index of illegitimate fertility (I_h) and of legitimate fertility (I_g).[g]

The importance of this observation is in what it implies with respect to the time trend in spread of voluntary birth control during the decline in illegitimacy. The rapid decline of marital fertility certainly implies that voluntary birth control was spreading through the population from the rather limited segments of societies who probably were using it before that.

The general demographic opinion has been that *coitus interruptus* was the main means of birth control at least in the initial decades of the European secular decline of marital fertility. There is increasing suspicion, however, that induced abortion also was used. As a means by which modern fertility declines have been achieved, Ryder says,

abortion has probably been significant always and everywhere. . . . The more we learn of the ineffectuality of most efforts at contraception, the more we are inclined to suspect a major covert role for abortion as a second line of defense against unwanted birth.[33]

Davis agrees. Referring to the high abortion rate in postwar Japan, Davis notes that:

Westerners profess to be astonished by this phenomenon, but they should not be. The behavior of the Japanese is essentially the same in kind as the behavior

---

[g]Ibid., p. 378. The I_g index is analogous to the I_h in that it compares the fertility of the population in question with the fertility of married Hutterite women of the same ages. An I_g of 600, for instance, indicates that the married women in that population were producing children at 60 percent the rate as did married Hutterite women of the same age categories.

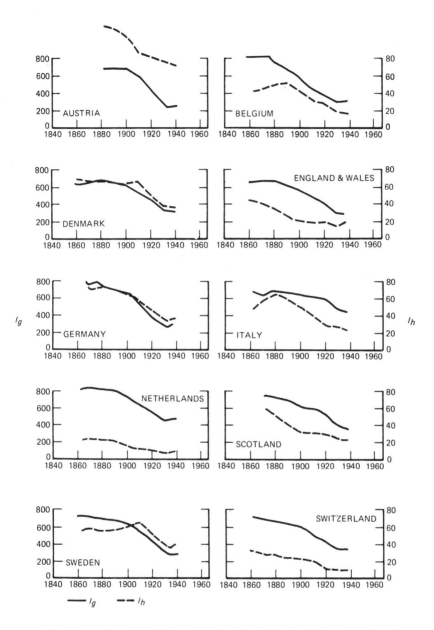

Figure 4-2. Indexes of Legitimate Fertility (I_g) and Illegitimate Fertility (I_h), Selected Countries of Europe, 1860-1940. Source: Shorter, Knodel, and Van de Walle, figure 2 (see note 13).

of West Europeans at a similar time in their social and demographic history. The main difference is that Japanese tolerance permits the abortion rate to be reasonably well known, whereas in the past of Europe the abortion rate has never been known and, for this reason, is usually ignored in population theory. . . . Yet there is indirect evidence that in the late nineteenth and early twentieth centuries in Western Europe abortion played a great role.[34]

On the basis of this and other evidence presented in their article, Shorter, Knodel, and Van de Walle conclude that "the decline of illegitimate fertility, as of legitimate fertility, has been to a very large extent the result of change in one of the intermediate variables, the use of contraception." This they say after having looked into changes in definition of marriage (which might help explain some regional differences), changes in the extent of nonmarital sexual activity, and changes in the likelihood of marriage occurring between conception and birth.[35]

The evidence is overwhelming that illegitimacy was reduced by means other than abstinence from intercourse throughout the period 1880 to 1940 in western Europe. But this does not necessarily imply that noncoitus still did not have an important role in preventing illegitimate fertility. Indeed, it could have remained the most important means of prevention, being supplemented increasingly by birth control throughout the period of fertility decline. It seems clear, nevertheless, that the normal assumption, that means of preventing illegitimate fertility other than avoiding nonmarital coitus are negligible, can be very misleading.

Europe Prior to 1880:
Two Case Studies

Our study of Europe 1850 to 1940 has allowed us to infer the contribution of voluntary birth control to the decline of illegitimacy. Left unanswered is the question: What happened to illegitimacy with the institution of late female marriage before the widespread use of voluntary birth control? This question is pertinent because most of the countries for which delayed marriage is now being advocated do not have widespread birth control (contraception or induced abortion). If we assume that birth control spread through the population of Europe from about 1880 to 1930, then we should try to find evidence for prior to 1880. Although systematic multinational evidence is lacking, we do have two provocative case studies by John Knodel, the first on the German states and the second on a Bavarian town.[36]

Responding partially to Malthusian ideas, in about the 1830s, a third of the German states instituted regulations that had the effect of delaying marriage. In those states, the regulations generally required that the groom produce evidence of having sufficient wealth or property, a secure income, or assured stable employment opportunities before he would be given permission to marry; in some states there was even a stated minimum age. Although these rules were *instituted* before data collections systems were prevalent, there are sound data to trace what happened when the restrictions were *relaxed* in the 1860s. Interestingly, records of the debate preceding the repeals clearly show that a major reason given was the supposed causal relation between legally forced delayed marriage and high illegitimacy rates. Knodel documents what must have been known to the legislators, that illegitimacy rates were higher in those states where marriage restrictions prevailed than in those in which marriage was not so restricted. This conclusion then was supported by the fact that the subsequent decline in illegitimacy was greater in those states which had had legally delayed marriage then repealed it than in states which had not legally delayed marriage in the first place.

Knodel followed this with a case study of a particular Bavarian village, Anhausen, near Augsburg, for which he found a village genealogy covering couples married between 1692 and 1939. The longer time span of these data allowed him to document not only the decline in illegitimacy with the relaxing of the marriage-delaying laws, as above, but also to register the earlier increase in illegitimacy with the institution of those laws. It serves to confirm his conclusion drawn from his earlier study of the German states.

A glance at Figure 4-2 reminds us that illegitimacy was particularly high in Austria and Germany in comparison with most other European countries in the mid-1800s, thus Anhausen may represent an extreme case. Unfortunately, we do not seem to have the data for a more extensive study of the relation between changes in illegitimacy and changes in age at marriage prior to the mid-1800s. The problem apparently is more with tracing nuptiality changes than with tracing illegitimacy changes. Regarding illegitimacy, Shorter, Knodel, and Van de Walle, confidently assert:

Around the middle of the eighteenth century a great secular increase in illegitimacy began all over Europe. In community after community for which parish register data are available, the proportion of illegitimate births increased rapidly.... The rise continued until around the middle of the nineteenth century."[37]

Regarding age at marriage, although Hajnal asserts that the "European pattern" had its origins before this period, it is not yet clear whether the late-marriage norm did spread progressively through the various segments of the European populations during the time when general illegitimacy also was rising.

Theoretical Discussion

The theme of the chapter so far has been negative. We have attempted to question the assumption of negligible illegitimacy in times of late marriage and of coital avoidance as the sole path for preventing birth with late marriage. If the reader has reached this point with a more skeptical view of those matters, then it is time to attempt a more positive formulation. We take this as our orienting question: Under what conditions is a high proportion of women nonmarried in the reproductive ages associated with high illegitimacy rates?

All of the following conditions must be met in order that a given woman produce one or more illegitimate births in her lifetime.

1. The number of years spent nonmarried but in the reproductive ages must be greater than zero.
2. Her coital frequency during those nonmarried years must be greater than zero.
3. In the period during which she has a coital frequency greater than zero, conception must be possible. For instance, she cannot be sterile. Nor can she be contracepting perfectly.
4. If and when she conceives, foetal mortality cannot be complete. For instance, she cannot induce abortion of all her pregnancies. Nor can she be incapable of carrying pregnancy safely to term.
5. Marriage cannot occur between conception and birth for all those pregnancies not ending in foetal mortality.

The reader will recognize that this list of conditions is suggested by the Davis-Blake list of intermediate variables between culture and fertility, treated in Chapter 3.[h]

To the degree that any of the five conditions is not met, the number of illegitimate births to the woman in her lifetime will be reduced. That is, the conditions represent substitutable means of reducing illegitimate births.

Moreover, to the degree that any one of the conditions is not met, the potential effect on illegitimacy of other conditions not being met is reduced. For instance, if the woman marries at the beginning of her reproductive years and stays married throughout them, thus failing condition 1, then there is not a possibility of illegitimate birth left for the other factors to control. For another instance, if she remains unmarried to age twenty-five but is kept cloistered away from men until marriage, then again there is no control being exercised by the other factors. For a final example, if all conceptions to her when she is nonmarried will end in induced abortion, then the influence of her nonmarriage, coital frequency, and fecundity on her number of illegitimate births will be redundant.

Thus we can say that the more of her years (in the reproductive ages) a woman spends nonmarried the greater the number of illegitimate births she will produce, to the degree that all of the following conditions prevail: Her coital frequency during the nonmarried years exceeds zero; her probability of conception per coitus exceeds zero; her probability of successful parturition per pregnancy exceeds zero; her probability of marriage between conception and birth is less than unity.

The same point can be stated on the aggregate level. The greater the proportion of woman years (within the reproductive period) spent nonmarried, the greater the number of illegitimate births per woman, to the degree that all of the following conditions prevail:

---

[h]In this approach we are following a path parallel to that of Philips Cutright in his analysis of the causes of illegitimacy, Cutright, "Illegitimacy," pp. 26-27, and also that of Shirley Foster Hartley, "From the 'Principle of Illegitimacy' to a Concatenated Theory of Illegitimacy" (Paper delivered at the Seventh World Conference of the International Sociological Association, Varna, Bulgaria, September, 1970). The definition of illegitimate birth employed does not include illegitimate births to women married at the time of the births. Shorter, Knodel, and Van de Walle, "Decline of Non-Marital Fertility in Europe," footnote 12.

48

Coital frequency during the nonmarried years exceeds zero; probability of conception from coitus exceeds zero; probability of successful parturition exceeds zero; and the probability of marriage between nonmarried conception and birth is less than unity.

Then under what conditions does being nonmarried not prevent fertility? Under the conditions that coital frequency of nonmarried women is high and that probability of conception per coitus is high and that probability of marriage between conception and live birth is low. But the relaxing of any of these conditions reduces the tendency of more nonmarriage to result in more illegitimacy. By implication a society raising its female age at marriage can reduce consequent rise in illegitimacy (1) by preventing coitus for unmarried women, and/or (2) by fostering contraception by unmarried women and/or (3) by fostering induced abortion by unmarried women.[i]

Policy Implications

For simplicity, let us confine our attention to the nuptiality policy most frequently advocated as a means to control fertility, delaying the female age at first marriage. Thus we will be dealing with the prospect of increase in the proportions of women nonmarried especially in the young years, say 15-24.

As a direct effect, a delay in the national female age at first marriage would tend to result in increased national levels of illegitimacy. The degree to which this tendency would be blocked would depend upon the capacity of the society to offset it by influencing the behavior of unmarried women. One class of nations in which illegitimacy would be relatively unlikely to rise with female age at marriage would be those nations in which voluntary birth control already is most widespread, both within and without marriages, that is, the technologically developed countries.

Another class of nations where illegitimacy might be relatively contained would be those in which premarital coital frequency, with or without contraception, can be controlled. One subclass might be a

---

[i]To be complete, we should add that a society raising its female age at marriage can limit its consequent rise in illegitimacy (4) by requiring marriage of all premaritally pregnant women before they give birth. However, there is a disturbing contradiction in such a suggestion since the requirement would itself limit raising the female age at marriage.

totalitarian nation, such as Communist China, where social controls supposedly are complete enough to ensure mass abstinence from premarital sex even with delayed marriage, though evidence is very thin.

Another subclass might be a society in which the extended residential family system is strong enough to assure sexual isolation of unmarried daughters until more advanced ages. But it is problematic whether even societies in which the extended family of residence and isolation of daughters is the norm (for example, Moslem societies) would be able to maintain those norms under the circumstance of daughters spending several more unmarried years in the household. Empirically, it seems that those societies with isolation of unmarried daughters in generationally-extended family households also are those in which women tend to be married very early.

If the above conclusions are correct, then the prospect is unpromising for most of the present nontotalitarian technologically underdeveloped countries. An abrupt increase in the present age of women at first marriages is likely to be closely associated with a rise in illegitimacy, because at present those countries are not characterized by widespread voluntary birth control or means for strongly controlling premarital coitus throughout youth.

Indeed, the one large-scale contemporary case we do have of the late age at first marriage in countries where birth control is not widespread is that of Latin America. In general, levels of illegitimacy are indeed high, partially as the result of consensual unions.[j] Latin America provides an excellent set of cases for future verification or refutation of the points being made here.

There are Asian countries in which there has been a rapid nuptiality transition away from the Asian type to an approximation of the European type. Aside from Japan, Korea is the most striking example, with Hong Kong, Taiwan, Singapore, and Ceylon less so.[38] It is notable, however, that these same countries would be chosen as illustrations of rapid recent spread of birth control. Moreover, I know of no analysis of illegitimacy trends in those countries during

[j]To quote Shirley Foster Hartley, a ranking of contemporary countries in terms of illegitimacy ratios shows "a rough geographical pattern with the highest ratios concentrated in the Central American and Caribbean countries followed by the South American nations." In Shirley Foster Hartley, "Contributions for Illegitimate and Premaritally Conceived Legitimate Births to Total Fertility," *Social Biology* 18 (June 1971): 179.

the nuptiality changes. Careful research in these countries might produce another valuable empirical test.

We have focused on the likely direct effects on illegitimacy of increasing age at first marriage, but illegitimacy is of secondary importance to those advocating the policy. While illegitimacy may rise with delayed marriage, on the other hand, overall fertility (illegitimate and legitimate) almost certainly would decline. That is, no matter how poor the control over the sexual behavior of unmarried young women, they are unlikely to achieve nonmaritally the level of fertility they would have experienced had they been married during those same years. To say that the rise in illegitimacy might be a subject of concern to policymakers is not to say that the rise in illegitimate fertility is likely to be so great as to balance the decline in legitimate fertility.

The point is rather that the potential rise in illegitimate fertility is minimized and the drop in total fertility is maximized along with delay in female marriage by instituting voluntary birth control or controlling premarital coitus. If one is pessimistic about controlling premarital coitus along with delayed marriage, then clearly the degree to which socially undesirable effects (illegitimacy) are minimized and socially desirable effects are maximized (reduction of total fertility) depends upon the degree of voluntary birth control by unmarried women.

In short, the effectiveness of a policy of delaying female age at marriage depends on voluntary birth control.[k]

Summary

Two assumptions normally are made by those either estimating the effect on fertility of delayed marriage or advocating delayed marriage as a policy for fertility reduction; that illegitimate fertility would remain negligible and that the main means by which nonmarriage would prevent fertility would be by reducing coital frequency of young women. The origins of these assumptions can be found in the advocacy by Thomas Malthus of delayed marriage as a morally acceptable alternative to voluntary birth control.

---

[k]These policy implications are discussed more fully in combination with others in Chapter 7.

Gathering the evidence regarding the first assumption, that illegitimate fertility would remain negligible with late female marriage, involves conceptual problems in defining illegitimacy. Accepting legal definitions of marriage results in defining births to consensual unions as illegitimate, no matter how durable and sanctioned by nongovernment agencies those unions might be. On the other hand, accepting, as legitimate, births from pregnancies which started before marriage might result in an underestimation of illegitimacy for some purposes. Nevertheless, using the legal definition of illegitimacy seems appropriate in assessing the possible effects of a government policy aimed at delaying legal marriage.

Gathering evidence relevant to the second assumption, regarding the means by which delayed marriage would result in reduced fertility, would have to be indirect. Lacking probable direct evidence on changes in coital frequency, one would rely on evidence of other methods being generally used by married women, such as contraception or induced abortion. Widespread marital use of birth control techniques would be presumptive evidence that the techniques probably were available to nonmarried women as well and that they could have been used to supplement abstinence from coitus in avoiding illegitimate fertility.

The two assumptions are evaluated in the case of western Europe 1850 to 1940, a period during which average female ages at marriage remained relatively late. Illegitimacy levels were highest at the beginning of this span, generally between 2 and 8 percent of the fertility that these women would have experienced had they behaved like married Hutterite women of the same age but undoubtedly somewhat larger in comparison with the more modest fertility they would have experienced as married western European women of the same age. There is partial evidence that these levels of illegitimacy prevailed when some voluntary birth control already was in use in Europe. There is stronger evidence that the decline of illegitimate fertility from 1850 through the 1930s paralleled the decline in marital fertility, brought about by increasing usage of birth control, contraception probably supplemented by induced abortion. Thus the assumptions that illegitimacy was avoided by avoiding coitus seems an oversimplification; progressively coital avoidance was supplemented by birth control in this role as illegitimacy was brought down to modern prewar European levels.

The conditions under which delayed marriage is most likely to be associated with illegitimacy can be logically deduced from the Davis-Blake analytical framework: under the conditions that coital frequency of nonmarried women is high and that the probability of conception per coitus is high and that the probability of livebirth per conception is high and that the probability of marriage between conception and live birth is low. Relaxing any one of these conditions reduces the tendency for delay in marriage to result in illegitimacy.

One policy implication of this deduction is that illegitimacy is likely to result from delayed marriage precisely in that class of countries for whom delayed marriage is most advocated as a suppressant of fertility; countries in which present female age at marriage is early and in which voluntary birth control is not widespread. Thus, if illegitimacy is to be held in check while fertility is reduced by delaying marriage, marriage delay would have to be accompanied by spread of birth control. Thus the two policies are seen not as alternatives but as logically combined.

5

Cohort Marital Status and Marital Dissolution

With this chapter we move one step further back in the causal chain leading from marital events to period fertility. Here, and in the next chapter, we treat cohort marital status as the dependent variable and marital events as independent variables. This chapter is devoted to the event of marital dissolution, voluntary or involuntary, and to the counteracting event of remarriage.

Our guiding question is: How effective has marital dissolution been in the past, and how effective is it likely to be in the future, in keeping women nonmarried, especially during their twenties?

Widowhood: Age Patterns

The event of a husband's death affects his wife's fertility potential by changing her status to that of widowed. This effect can be cancelled, sooner or later, by another event: widow remarriage. Thus we are interested in the net effect of the two events of husband death and widow remarriage in determining how long the woman remains in the status of widowed.

Since our focus is on how widowhood influences cohort marital status, we should represent widowhood from a cohort perspective.[a] Unfortunately, the most generally available and reliable information on widowed status is from national censuses, and they present data not longitudinally for cohorts but cross-sectionally for the day of the census. This should not be an insurmountable handicap, however, if we pretend that the cross-sectional data for a series of

---

[a]Ideal data for a cohort analysis of widowhood, and divorce, would be full marital histories of all survivors of specified female birth cohorts, recording times of events affecting widowed or divorced status. Census data conventionally record present marital statuses defined in terms of the most recent event, and thus represent truncated histories. Fertility surveys, a promising new source of retrospective data, however, usually include only presently-married women in their samples.

cohorts represents the history of an hypothetical cohort, and allow for recent time trends.[b]

Table 5-1 and Figure 5-1 present, for each of three countries at recent dates, a series of seven percentages, one each for the female age categories 15-19 through 45-49. The seven percentages can be thought of as the history of an hypothetical cohort. Viewed longitudinally, each percentage has as its numerator the woman-years spent in widowed status and as its denominator the total woman-years lived by the cohort in that age category. The larger the proportions, the greater the time "lost" to reproduction by means of widowhood.

We choose India and Sweden for Table 5-1 and Figure 5-1 because they represent extremely contrasting widowhood situations. India has had relatively high mortality and low widow remarriage; Sweden has had low mortality and easy remarriage. The United States is presented also, both because it is more familiar to many

Table 5-1
Percentage of Female Population Widowed, by Age, Recent Figures for India, United States, and Sweden

Age	India, 1961	U.S., 1967[a]	Sweden, 1965
15-19	0.5	0.1	0.0
20-24	1.3	0.3	0.1
25-29	2.9	0.4	0.3
30-34	6.4	1.2	0.6
35-39	11.2	2.7[b]	1.1
40-44	20.7		2.0
45-49	28.8		3.6

[a]Estimate
[b]Women aged 35-44.
Source: *Demographic Yearbook, 1968* (New York: United Nations, 1969), Table 7.

---

[b]Suppose all of the cohorts represented in the cross section had identical cohort marital status histories with respect to widowhood. Then one could combine successive age categories taken from different cohorts and still end up with the same cohort widowhood status history. Specifically, one could construct the widowhood status history of an hypothetical cohort by combining widowhood status for present age categories 15-19 through 45-49 as represented in a given census. This is an inaccurate representation of the widowhood status histories of some of the real cohorts involved only to the degree that these cohorts differed among themselves in widowhood status history.

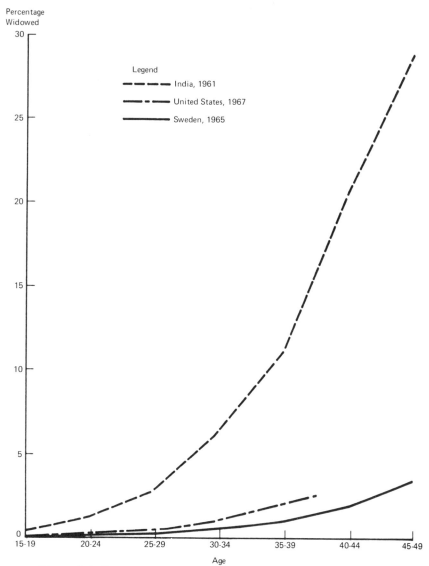

Figure 5-1. Percentage of Female Population Widowed, by Age, Recent Figures for India, United States, and Sweden. Source: table 5-1.

readers and because it represents an intermediate case of moderately low mortality and easy remarriage.

In all three countries the percentage widowed stays at a low level until the early thirties and then rises. Even in the case of India, the percentage widowed is still less than 3 percent in the age category 25-29 and only 6.5 percent in ages 30-34. Thus the age pattern of widowhood in these three countries is such as to have minimal impact upon the very years of the cohort marital history most relevant to fertility; the twenties and especially the early twenties. Although it is likely that our use of cross-sectional data exaggerates the age differences in widowhood by giving misleadingly large percentages for later ages, they would not be exaggerating the absolute smallness of values for the early ages.[c]

Widowhood: Trends and Prospects

Table 5-2 presents data on the time trends of widowhood for India and for Norway. These countries are taken as examples of countries where mortality has been high until recently (India) and where it had declined at an earlier time (Norway). They both show the worldwide trend during this century toward less widowhood.[d] Moreover, they

Table 5-2
Percentage of Female Population Widowed at Specified Ages, India and Norway Around 1900 and 1960

	India		Norway	
Age	1901	1961	1900	1960
30	18.5	6.4	2.1	0.5
35	25.8	11.2	3.5	0.9
40	40.2	20.7	5.8	1.4
45	46.4	28.9	9.1	3.1
50	63.2	45.5	13.3	5.7

Source: Bogue, p. 343 (see footnote d).

[c]Let us assume that any national time trend in the recent past is likely to be in the direction of less widowhood, due to less husband mortality not counterbalanced by less widow remarriage. Then the percentage widowed for the older age categories probably are overestimates of the widowhood that will be experienced by the women presently in the younger age categories. Thus the differences between the degree of cohort widowhood at younger as opposed to older ages may be somewhat exaggerated by using cross-sectional data. Nevertheless, use of cross-sectional data does not tend to underestimate the absolute degree of widowhood in the younger age categories.

[d]Bogue claims that this is a general trend and that his Table 11-6B contains numerous additional examples. Donald J. Bogue, *Principles of Demography* (New York: John Wiley & Sons, Inc., 1969), pp. 343-46.

show that the widowhood decline is occurring at all ages, perhaps especially at the younger ages. Thus the widowhood decline is not likely to alter the widowhood age pattern we observed in the preceding section.

If the proportion of fecund-aged women who were in the status of widowed has been decreasing generally, what are the prospects for a continuation of that trend? How confident can we be that the fertility import of widowed status will remain at its present low level or even lower? A guess about world widowhood prospects should be based on guesses about trends in the two events which initiate and terminate widowhood status: husband death and widow remarriage.

The general relationship between cohort mortality history and cohort widowhood history can be seen through an hypothetical example. Suppose we have two cohorts of women, both of which experience the same age schedule of first marriage rates and of remarriage rates, but which experience different age schedules of mortality rates, male and female. In the low-mortality cohort, of those ever-married women themselves surviving, a lower proportion will be widowed, because their husbands also would have suffered a lower mortality schedule. All else being equal, a lower general mortality means a lower proportion of survivors widowed. Eduardo Arriaga states it more formally.

As mortality decreases . . . the probability of survival for both men and women increases and, therefor, so does the number of unions. Since the probability of survival of unions is the product of the probabilities of survival for men and women, a decrease in mortality has more effect on the probability of joint survival than on each of its components. Thus the relative increase of unions will be larger than the relative increase of either men or women.[1]

Generally, mortality has been declining rapidly in the past and is likely to make some less rapid declines in the future. It is difficult to foresee the circumstances under which a sustained increase in mortality would again be tolerated as long as nations have the natural resources to avoid it. Therefore, on the basis of a presumed decline or stability in general mortality, we would expect no increase of husband mortality and the incidence of widowhood.

But there are complexities in the relationship between general mortality and husband mortality relevant to our problem of time trends. First is the greater likelihood of husbands dying than wives dying. This is partially due to the norm of husbands being older than their brides, thus constantly suffering the mortality rates of more advanced ages than their wives. In addition, male age-specific mortality tends to be higher than female age-specific mortality. A change so that husband mortality was the same or less than wife mortality would have the effect of decreasing the incidence of female widowhood at a given general mortality level.

What are the prospects especially for technologically underdeveloped countries? It is probable that underdeveloped countries in which female age at first marriage is now early will experience a decrease in age gap between husband and wife along with any secular trend toward later marriage, and this might tend to decrease the extent of husband mortality, especially at earlier female ages. However, according to Bogue, the higher age-specific mortality of males as contrasted with females tends to increase with the general decline in mortality, and this might increase the prospects of husband mortality with general mortality decline.[2] In short the two aspects would tend to counteract each other.

Second, the earlier the age at which a woman marries, the more likely she is to be widowed by a given age. This is a simple result of the forces of mortality having a longer duration in which to risk her marriage. Thus, everything else being equal, societies with normally late ages of women at first marriage would tend to have lower proportions of women widowed at early ages. If one makes the plausible assumption that age at first marriage for women is more likely to increase than to decrease in presently underdeveloped countries, then this factor would bring lower likelihood of female widowhood at given mortality levels.

Third, the proportion of women in widowed status at a given age depends on their ability to survive mortality themselves after their husbands have died. Widowhood can end either by remarriage or by death of the widow. If we follow Collver's inference, that widow mortality especially is high in underdeveloped countries, then technological development might bring better relative survival improvement for widows and thus a greater proportion of surviving women in the status of widowed.[3]

In sum, these complexities in the relationship between general mortality and the incidence of widowhood should not operate in such a way as to confound the direct impact of mortality on widowhood: as general mortality declines, the incidence of husband mortality and of widowhood also will decline.

However, our treatment so far has dealt only with the incidence of one of the events determining the prevalence of widowhood: husband death. The prevalence of widowhood is also affected by the incidence of widow remarriage. What are the trends and prospects for widow remarriage, especially in technologically underdeveloped countries? Our answers will have to be based primarily on ethnographic evidence.[e]

Davis and Blake hypothesize that bans on widow remarriage are likely to be strongest in societies where the joint household (including extended families) is strongest relative to either the larger clan or the smaller conjugal family. In these cultures, the sanctions against widow remarriage will be strong because of the awkwardness it would involve in kin relations, especially with respect to property. Where the clan is relatively strong, on the other hand, remarriage normally is prompt by such means as remarriage to the brother of the deceased husband.[4] Historically, India has been the extreme example of the joint-household pattern, and Davis has pointed out that the ban on widow remarriage might historically have helped to hold India's fertility in check.[5] This hypothesis is not universally accepted, but nevertheless we can spell out its implications.[6]

If most contemporary technologically underdeveloped countries have traditional cultures emphasizing the joint household and extended family rather than the clan, and if there is a general trend in these countries away from the dominance of the extended family and toward the dominance of conjugal family, as William Goode claims, then one would expect an increase in the likelihood of widow remarriage.[7] Bogue generalizes that this, in fact, is the case.

One of the outstanding indexes of modernization all over the world is the weakening of this cultural prohibition and the increased freedom of widowed or divorced persons to marry—irrespective of age.[8]

Indeed, Bogue claims that there is a general trend toward greater remarriage, even among industrial nations.

---

[e]Vital registration of marriage is especially incomplete and also lacking in detail about the previous marital history of the partners. Census data do not normally distinguish between persons in their first marital unions and those in later ones, and thus do not afford a simple method of inferring remarriage.

Our best guess about prospects for widowhood status seems clear: if husband death is likely either to stay stable or to decline, and if the probability of widow remarriage is likely to go up or at least stay stable, then the proportion of women widowed in the reproductive ages is likely at least to stay at its present low level and more probably to decline further.[f]

Divorce: Age Patterns

Our decision to use divorce alone to represent voluntary dissolution of marriage is arbitrary and may result in some underestimation of the effect of marital dissolution on cohort marital status. Divorce (which involves permission for remarriage) may be supplemented or replaced by legal separation (which does not permit remarriage) and/or by annulment (which states that the marriage never existed).[9] The underestimation is likely to be greatest in countries where the dominant religion forbids divorce, such as Catholic countries.[g] Therefore, the danger of underestimating the impact of marital dissolution will be minimized if we confine our attention temporarily to countries in which divorce is permitted.

Our interest is not in divorce and remarriage as events but rather in their net effect on cohort marital status by keeping women in the

---

[f]I have defended in Chapter 3 the contention that marital events influence fertility almost entirely by means of influencing cohort marital status. However, footnoted there were some complications in that picture, two of which can be illustrated by the case of the influence of widowhood on fertility.

First, it is possible that frequent widowing, not always followed by remarriage of women, may increase the probability of selectivity of wives on the basis of demonstrated fecundity. That is, potential husbands may select or reject from among available widows as partners on the basis of how many live births the widows have produced in their past marriages.

Second, it is possible that starting a new marriage, even with a previously married wife, starts a new round of childbearing which would have not occurred to that woman had she remained in the defunct marriage.

[g]The arguments against inclusion of legal separation in considering voluntary marital dissolution are as follows: (1) Our definition of a marital union is one in which coitus and reproduction are sanctioned. It is not universally clear whether legally-separated couples still are permitted to have sexual contact and to bear children, even though they are absolved from sexual responsibilities. (2) The distinction between legal separation and informal separation or desertion is vague and hard to draw with clarity adequate for comparative analysis. (3) Whereas the event of remarriage is recorded, however imperfectly, the event of reunion after separation normally is not; thus it is impossible to study both events involved in determining periods in legally-separated status.

status of divorced. As in our study of widowhood above, we will rely on census data for examples of generalizations about divorced status. These cross-sectional census data can be viewed cautiously as the histories of hypothetical cohorts.[h]

Table 5-3 and Figure 5-2 present data on the age pattern of divorce for contemporary India, United States, and Sweden. These countries were chosen partially because we already are familiar with the widowhood age pattern in them, from Table 5-1 and Figure 5-1. In addition they dramatize (perhaps exaggerate) the contrast between two very different but prevalent marital patterns, that of preindustrial Asia and that of the modern West. For each of the countries we present a series of percentages for the seven successive age periods of the supposed reproductive period, the percentages representing the proportion of the total woman-years which were spent in divorced status.

In India, the country with the lowest overall level of divorce, the proportion divorced (or separated) changes very little from one age category to the next. In contrast, for the United States and Sweden,

Table 5-3

Percentage of Female Population Divorced, by Age, Recent Figures for India, United States, and Sweden

Age	India, 1961[a]	U.S., 1967[b]	Sweden, 1965
15-19	0.6	0.2	0.0
20-24	0.9	1.8	0.5
25-29	1.0	3.3	2.1
30-34	1.0	4.5	3.2
35-39	1.0	4.7[c]	4.1
40-44	1.0		5.0
45-49	0.9		5.3

[a]Divorced and separated, rather than divorced only.

[b]Estimate, rather than census.

[c]Aged 35-44.

Source: *Demographic Yearbook, 1968* (New York: United Nations, 1969), Table 7.

---

[h]See note b for the rationale behind interpreting cross-sectional status data in longitudinal terms. We are not able to guess whether interpreting cross-sectional data in hypothetical-cohort terms has caused us to underestimate or overestimate the differences among the age categories. Arguments can be made in either direction.

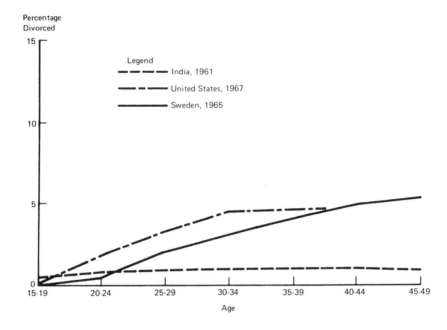

Figure 5-2. Percentage of Female Population Divorced, by Age, Recent Figures for India, United States, and Sweden. Source: table 5-3.

with higher general levels of divorce, the proportion divorced starts at a negligible level in the teens (probably due to small proportions ever-married in the teens), then rises continuously through the succeeding age categories of the supposedly reproductive period. Thus, to the degree that these countries are typical, "modern" higher proportions of women divorced are gathered especially in the later female age categories where they would have less negative impact upon fertility. Bogue claims that this pattern is indeed general:

Divorce reaches its maximum prevalence at the very end of the childbearing period, or even later. For this reason the effect on birthrates of divorce is comparatively minor. . . .[10]

However, to say that this age pattern has prevailed in the past and present does not necessarily give assurance that it will prevail in the future. To gain that assurance, it is necessary to look more closely at what must be causing the age pattern of divorced status, the age pattern of the relevant events: divorce, and remarriage of divorcees.

Let us contrast the age pattern of divorce with that of widowhood. Since there is a standard pattern of relative mortality by age, with annual mortality risk increasing slowly from childhood through adulthood, the annual likelihood of being widowed increases with age of woman. No such automatic increase in annual risk applies to divorce. In the United States, at least, divorce seems to be spread over all marriage durations fairly evenly, although there is a slightly greater divorce risk during the first couple years after marriage than in later years.[11] Thus the age pattern of the initiating event is somewhat different for divorce in contrast with widowhood, and likely to remain so.

Explanation for the higher proportions in divorced status at later ages is more likely to be found in the age patterns of remarriage than in the age pattern of divorce. For one thing, divorced women generally have a very high likelihood of being remarried. It is generally higher, for instance, than for widowed women. For another thing, remarriage is more likely for women divorced at young ages than for women divorced at older ages.[12] It seems plausible, then, that the main reason for so few woman years in the younger ages being spent in divorced status in contrast with the older ages, is not that divorce and separation are less likely then, but that women are likely to remarry more rapidly after young divorces.[i]

There seems no reason for doubting that this same age pattern of divorced status will prevail in the future as divorce levels either rise or stabilize at high levels. For, as we shall see below, a rise in the incidence of remarriage is closely associated with a rise in the incidence of divorce.

---

[i]The age pattern of widowhood observed above also could be caused partially by greater likelihood of rapid remarriage by young widows in contrast with older widows. In the case of widowhood, the age pattern of husbands' death and the age pattern of remarriage probably complement each other in producing a pattern of increasing widowhood status with age. In the case of divorce, on the other hand, the age pattern of remarriage is the dominant, if not the sole, factor causing the age pattern of increasing divorced status with age.

Divorce: Trends and Prospects

If one assumes a general trend toward technological development on something like the western model in the world, then the prospects are for a general rise in the incidence of divorce in the world. William Goode detailed this position in his classic work *World Revolution and Family Patterns* in 1963.[13] Let us detail some of the past time trends which brought Goode to this position.

In general, preindustrial societies have lower divorce rates than modern Western societies. There are notable exceptions to this generalization: traditional Moslem nations, Japan in the decades before 1920, some matrilineal tribes in sub-Saharan Africa.[14] And in these exceptions, technological development may even bring a decrease in divorce, according to Goode. But the more normal preindustrial situation is better illustrated by, say, contemporary India or preindustrial Europe.

The long-term secular trend in Western divorce rates at least from the mid-1800s to the present is clearly upward, and the United States serves as an extreme example of the trend.[15] Carter and Glick summarize the rise in U.S. rates from 1890 to 1960: "During this 70-year period, there was a three-fold increase in the rate of divorce, with most of the rise taking place during the first 30 years."[16] There have been deviations from the secular trend in the United States; a decline during the depression, a surge immediately after World War II, a stabilization for a decade after the surge. But the most recent evidence indicates a continuation of the long-term rise.[17]

The expectation that such a rise in divorce will be a feature of continued technological development both in the West and in westernizing nations is based on more sophisticated reasoning than a blind projection of past trends into the future. Both William Goode and Bernard Farber have developed theoretical positions which support this conclusion. Goode says that emphasis on the conjugal unit, rather than the extended kinship unit, is functional in industrial economies. A feature of the conjugal emphasis is freedom to change partners.[18] Farber says that with the decline in the extended-kin concern for orderly replacement of the family over time comes the acceptance of universal and permanent availability of adult men and women for marriage and remarriage.[19]

But an increase in the incidence of divorce does not necessarily mean an equivalent increase in the prevalence of divorced status. It is theoretically possible for increased incidence of divorce to be offset by an increased incidence of remarriage.

Indeed, there are good reasons for expecting a rise in divorce to be associated with a rise in remarriage. Empirically this has been so.[20] And, upon reflection, the association seems almost tautological: the definition of divorce itself includes the permission for remarriage. One could even make a case that the prospect of easy remarriage is a necessary condition for a high incidence of divorce.

The United States provides an example of how female remarriage operates in a society with high incidence of divorce. Remarriage rates are higher for divorced women than for either widowed women or than (marriage rates) for unmarried women, and especially high for young divorcees. Divorced women aged 14-24 have better than a fifty-fifty chance of being remarried each year. Over the whole reproductive span, age 14-44, the yearly chances of remarriage are one in five.[21]

If divorce and remarriage are so closely linked, then divorced status becomes a transitional status. The proportion of women in a society divorced depends upon how swiftly and completely women switch from one marriage to the next. What will be the time trends in female divorced status in the future? On the one hand, increased incidence of divorce would put more women into the "transitional" divorced status at any given time. On the other hand, greater incidence of divorce might indirectly speed the transition from one marriage to another, by such means as simplifying the legal work and/or increasing the size of the supply of potential partners for remarriage. In short, the net result is theoretically problematical.

However, we do have some empirical evidence of time trends in female divorced status from the U.S. This country is pertinent because it is an extreme example of the trends in incidence of divorce and remarriage cited above. Carter and Glick supply proportions of women aged fourteen and over who were in divorced status. The proportion was 0.4 percent in 1890, 1.6 percent in 1940, and 3.1 percent in 1965.[22] Even more recently, the U.S. Census Bureau reports that "there were 42 currently divorced women for every 1,000 women with husband present in 1960 as compared with 66 per 1,000 in 1972."[23] So the trend is slowly upward. But the proportions still are small, and would be even smaller for women in the earlier, most reproductive ages.

Widowhood and Divorce Combined

So far we have been dealing with the age patterns, trends, and prospects for widowhood and for divorce separately. It is in their combined effect on nonmarried status that we ultimately are interested. This is particularly important to assess since we have seen that widowhood and divorce move in contrasting patterns with major social changes.

First let us look at the age pattern for the combined statuses of widowed and divorced. These are shown in Table 5-4 and Figure 5-3, for India, Sweden, and the United States—countries chosen to represent divergent combinations of widowhood and divorce. A first observation from the table is that in all three countries there is a net increase in the proportion of women nonmarried with age, for reasons of widowhood and divorce combined. The proportions nonmarried are particularly low during the ages 20-24 and 25-29, the ages of special import to fertility. Thus even if one makes the plausible assumption that with modernization countries will become less like India and more like Sweden in terms of divorce and

Table 5-4
Percentage of Female Population Widowed or Divorced, by Age, Recent Figures for India, United States, and Sweden

Age	India, 1961[a]	U.S., 1967[b]	Sweden, 1965
15-19	1.2	0.2	0.0
20-24	2.2	2.1	0.6
25-29	3.9	3.7	2.4
30-34	7.5	5.7	3.8
35-39	12.2		5.2
40-44	21.7	7.4[c]	7.0
45-49	29.7		8.9

[a]Divorced and separated, rather than divorced only.

[b]Estimate, rather than census.

[c]Age 35-44.

Source: *Demographic Yearbook, 1968* (New York: United Nations, 1969), Table 7.

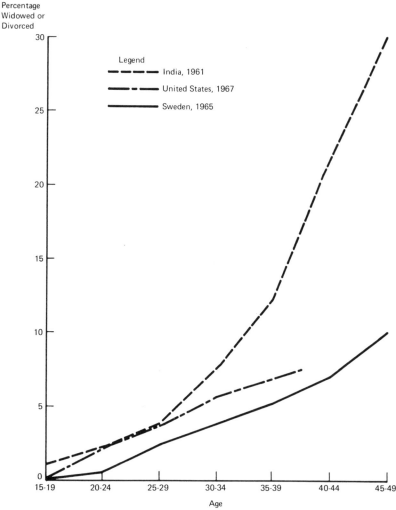

Figure 5-3. Percentage of Female Population Widowed or Divorced, by Age, Recent Figures for India, United States, and Sweden. Source: table 5-4.

mortality behavior, the relative unimportance of these influences on the younger women will remain.

Although this conclusion is based on cross-sectional data, it is supported by an unusual case study based on cohort analysis of survey data of San Jose, Costa Rica. Onaka and Yaukey analyzed retrospective marital histories for a sample of all women in San Jose and computed the percentage of the reproductive time lost, by age, as a combined result of widowhood, divorce, and separation. Table 5-5 is taken from that analysis.[24] The results are the more noteworthy because they happen to refer to a type of nation whom we have been avoiding in our analysis because of conceptual and technical difficulties, a Catholic nation with widespread consensual unions. Yet the same general age pattern of nonmarriage appears here even when one includes consensual unions as marital ones, even where there are sanctions against divorce, and even when one includes the effects of "separation."

We choose to use the United States as an example in tracing the time trends in the combined effects of widowhood and divorce. It probably represents a case for maximal proportion nonmarried because of dissolution in a modern nation, a case of very high divorce, and only moderately low widowhood. For emphasis and for simplicity, we have chosen to present proportions only for the very fertile female ages 20-24 and 25-29.

The proportion nonmarried because of widowhood and divorce combined has remained essentially stable from 1890 through 1960 for both age categories of women. There have been ups and downs during the period, but no overall time trend of any great magnitude. Clearly this stability in net effect represents a balance between a lowering proportion widowed and a rising proportion divorced. In the United States, this balance apparently has been almost perfect.

Table 5-5
Percentage of Reproductive Time Lost to Women, by Age, Because of Widowhood, Divorce, and Separation, San Jose, Costa Rica, 1964

Age	Percent Time Lost[a]
15-19	2.7
20-24	6.1
25-29	7.6
30-34	12.2
35-39	16.0
40-44	18.7
45-49	21.3

[a]Number of cases = 1,226.

Source: Onaka and Yaukey (see note 24).

Table 5-6

Percentage of Young Female Population Widowed or Divorced, United States, 1890 to 1960

Year	Aged 20-24			Aged 25-29		
	Widowed	Divorced	Widowed, Divorced	Widowed	Divorced	Widowed, Divorced
1960	0.3	1.8	2.1	0.7	2.6	3.3
1950	0.4	1.7	2.1	0.9	2.5	3.4
1940	0.6	0.9	1.5	1.3	1.8	3.1
1930	1.0	1.1	2.1	2.1	1.8	3.9
1920	1.4	0.6	2.0	2.6	0.9	3.5
1910	1.2	0.5	1.7	2.4	0.7	3.1
1900	1.4	0.4	1.8	2.9	0.6	3.5
1890	1.2	0.2	1.4	2.8	0.4	3.2

Source: *U.S. Census of Population, 1960: Detailed Characteristics, U.S. Summary,* Table 177.

Summary

With the present chapter, our attention turned from the effects of cohort marital status to the determinants of cohort marital status. Specifically, the present chapter deals with involuntary and voluntary marital dissolution as determinants of cohort marital status.

The prevalence of women in the status of widowed in a given age category is determined by the incidences of two balancing processes—husband mortality and widow remarriage. The net effect of these two processes normally is to produce an age pattern of widowhood with the prevalence lowest at the younger, more fertile, female ages. Moreover, recent time trends of widowhood prevalence seem to be downward internationally.

If present social trends continue, the prevalence of widowhood during female reproductive years is likely either to be stable or, more likely, to decline further in the future. Continuing advances against mortality are the main basis for this prediction. Nevertheless, the effect of this trend may be complicated, by changes in relative ages of husbands and wives, changes in the relative age-specific mortality levels of husbands and wives, changes in the normal age at marriage and duration of risk of husband mortality, and changes in mortality of widows relative to that of married women of the same age.

Voluntary marital dissolution, best represented for our purposes by divorce, follows quite a different pattern from widowhood. There may be no standard age pattern for the prevalence of divorced status, as there was for widowed status, because the age of divorce is not so clearly a factor of age as is husband's death. It appeared in our examples that countries with higher rates of divorce were more likely to have patterns of lower proportions in divorced status in the younger female reproductive ages than in older reproductive ages, probably due to the greater rapidity of remarriage of young divorcees.

The general association of technological development with high incidence of divorce has been well documented and incorporated in theory by William Goode and others. However, both observed past trends and the ones predicted by theory for the future specify an increase not only in divorce but also in remarriage. Thus the prospects with respect to the net effect of these two, that is, the proportions in the interim status of divorced, is problematical. For instance, the increase in the proportion divorced at the crucial young female reproductive ages in the United States has been shown to increase only gradually over the last seventy-five years.

The effects of divorce and widowhood combine in complex ways. Since their age patterns of prevalence are generally similar, the age pattern of widowed *and* divorced status is one of increasing prevalence with increasing age, leaving only 4 percent or fewer of women in their twenties nonmarried for those reasons in the typical countries we studied. On the other hand, the likely downward trend in widowhood and possible upward trend in divorced status will balance in ways difficult to predict. In the case of the United States, they almost balanced each other over the past decades.

The implication for fertility is clear. Divorce and widowhood combined tend to keep only small proportions of women nonmarried during those years when they would have been most fertile, in their twenties. Therefore, they do little to suppress fertility. Moreover, there is no prospect for much change toward increased fertility suppression through divorce and widowhood along with secular trends toward modernization.

All of our guesses about the future for divorce and widowhood, however, presume no new kind of intervention by governments to alter the patterns. In fact, however, divorce and remarriage might be particularly susceptible to government policies. This point is elaborated in Chapter 7.

Cohort Marital Status and First Marriage

The only events which can determine the marital-status history of the survivors of a cohort of women are first marriage, widowhood, divorce, and remarriage. Of these, the event which normally has most ultimate impact upon fertility is first marriage, a point underlined in our initial section titled "Age Patterns of Single Status."

If the first-marriage process is deemed so important for cohort marital status and thus fertility, then we need a better understanding of the social and demographic determinants of the first-marriage process. Summarizing our knowledge on that topic is beyond the scope of the present book, although I hope to undertake it later. What this chapter offers is background for such an undertaking, a description of the nature of the first-marriage process followed by an identification of the basic variables in that process.

Let us adopt some simplifying vocabulary for the chapter. *Cohort single status* will mean female cohort marital status with respect to the proportion *never-married* for a series of age categories from 15 through 49. *Marriage* events are taken to mean only *first* marriage; not to include remarriages. *Nuptiality* is taken to mean the first-marriage process; not to include remarriage.

Age Patterns of Single Status

Table 6-1 and Figure 6-1 present the percentages single for seven successive age classes of women according to recent cross-sectional data from India, the United States, and Sweden. The three countries were chosen for illustration because they represent contrasting first-marriage patterns and because they may be familiar to the reader from Chapter 5. Since they present cross-sectional data rather than cohort data, the table and figure give only an approximation of

Table 6-1

Percentage of Female Population Single, by Age, Recent Figures for India, United States, and Sweden

Age	India, 1961	U.S., 1967[a]	Sweden, 1965
15-19	29.2	87.8	96.2
20-24	6.0	32.8	57.4
25-29	1.9	9.9	20.2
30-34	1.0	4.7	10.8
35-39	0.7	4.7[b]	8.6
40-44	0.6		8.5
45-49	0.5		8.6

[a]Estimate, rather than census.

[b]Age 35-44.

Source: *Demographic Yearbook, 1968* (New York: United Nations, 1969), Table 7.

the history of any actual cohort of women.[a,b] Nevertheless, two points emerge.

The first point is that the woman-years spent single tend to be the youngest "reproductive" years and thus to include the most fecund years. The proportions single start at their highest in the age category 15-19 then stabilize with the age class 35-39. True, the high

[a]That approximation would be close if marital patterns had been stable over the fertile periods of the whole series of female cohorts represented in the cross sections, but that is unlikely. On the one hand, if we assume a "marriage boom" in the Western countries immediately after World War II and through the 1950s, then the younger age classes for the United States and Sweden are likely to have smaller proportions single as they reach more advanced ages than is implied by Table 6-1. On the other hand, if we assume that the trend is toward later age at marriage in India, then the women currently aged 15-19 are likely to have larger proportions single in age classes 20-24 or 25-29 than is implied by the table. That is, the difference between younger and older age classes of women in actual cohorts is likely to be overestimated for the United States and Sweden and to be underestimated for India. John Hajnal, "The Marriage Boom," *Population Index* 19 (April 1953): 80-101. S.N. Agarwala, *Age at Marriage in India* (Allahabad, India: Kitab Mahal Private, Ltd., 1962), pp. 69-82.

[b]There is a secondary source of error in using cross-sectional data on single status to represent cohort single status: marital-status differentials in mortality or in net migration. Single women (vs. ever-married women) may have different rates of mortality or migration and that may influence their relative likelihood of surviving and being present to be enumerated in censuses. Moreover, since older women are likely to have had longer periods since their first marriages for these differential processes to operate, the age patterns of single status may be influenced as well as the overall levels. However, mortality and migration differentials probably are unimportant on the national level. John Hajnal, "Age at Marriage and Proportions Marrying," *Population Studies* 7 (November 1953), Appendix II, pp. 127-29. Agarwala, *Age at Marriage*, Chapter 2, pp. 6-23.

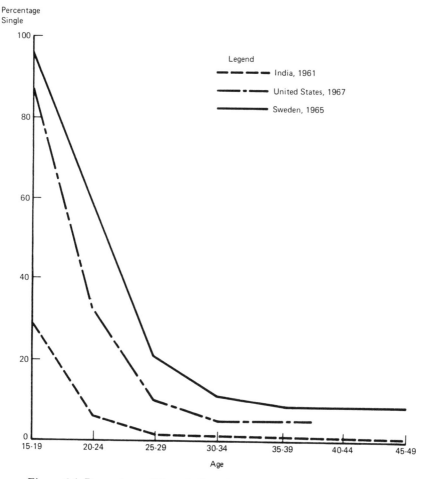

Percentage
Single

Legend

― ― ― ― India, 1961

―――•――― United States, 1967

――――― Sweden, 1965

Age

Figure 6-1. Percentage of Female Population Single, by Age, Recent Figures for India, United States, and Sweden. Source: table 6-1.

proportion single in the age class 15-19 may not have much impact on fertility because of adolescent subfecundity. Nevertheless, the age category in which single status is next most prevalent is the 20-24 category, one which we have pointed out as crucial for period fertility not only because of its high fecundity but also because of its importance in determining age of women at childbearing.[1]

The second point is that in the early twenties failure to have a first marriage normally puts a large proportion of women out of the married status, much larger than the combined forces of widowhood and divorce. Referring back to Table 5-4, we find that even in India for the age class 20-24 the proportion single is 2.7 times as great as the proportion in widowed and divorced statuses combined. The equivalent ratios for the United States and Sweden are 15.6 and 95.7, respectively. In the two Western countries represented—the United States and Sweden—the proportions still single in the important age category 20-24 is about one-third to one-half of the women.

Cohort Single Status and the First-Marriage Process

The form of the age curve of proportions single found in Figure 6-1 is dictated by the nature of the marriage process. Universally, cohort proportions single start highest at the youngest ages and decrease until the last member of the cohort who ever is to marry has married.[c] The following two aspects of the first-marriage process dictate such a curve: (1) all members of the cohort enter the status of single simultaneously at birth; (2) members leave the status of single serially over time, according to a schedule of age-specific rates of first marriage.

Thus the determinants of single status are different from the determinants of widowhood and divorce, treated in Chapter 5. In both of those processes, the initiation to the status of widowed or divorced was not simultaneous nor universal but rather serial and incomplete according to a schedule of rates. Thus the proportions widowed or divorced were determined by balances between the processes of entering (via husband's death or divorce) and leaving (via remarriage) the status. In contrast, in dealing with the first-marriage process we need not think of the process of entering as a variable.

Indeed, the process of first marriage bears a close resemblance to the process of death. The same simultaneous, universal event, birth, initiates a cohort both into the status of single and into the status of living. Both nuptiality and mortality deplete the ranks in the initial

---

[c]Ansley Coale recently has pointed out (a) the similarities in form and (b) the dimensions of variation among curves describing proportions ever-married for cohorts. The proportions ever-married is, of course, the complement of proportion single. Ansley J. Coale, "Age Patterns of Marriage," *Population Studies* 25 (July 1971): 193-96.

statuses by attrition according to an age schedule of rates, changing their status to ever-married (in the case of nuptiality) or to dead (in the case of mortality). The sole relevant formal difference between the processes is that all members of a cohort eventually die, but not all members of a cohort necessarily ever marry.

The technical advantage gained by making the analogy between first marriage and death is substantial. Demographers have been studying mortality for much longer than they have nuptiality and the mortality models they have developed are sophisticated. If the same models can be adapted to describe nuptiality, then much effort will have been saved. That actually has been done in the case of the most useful mortality model of all: The *life table* model has been adapted to produce *nuptiality tables*.[2]

For examples, we present in Table 6-2 selected columns from nuptiality tables for United States white vs. nonwhite women, average figures for the decade 1950 to 1960.[d,e]

The n_x column simply states the schedule of nuptiality rates by age, the probability of being first married between age x and age $x + 1$.[f] The N_x column shows what n_x implies with respect to the depletion in the ranks of the single by stating, for each age x, the number of women still single from an hypothetical set of 100,000 original women. Column M_x was derived by multiplying nuptiality rates (n_x) against women still single at a given birthday (N_x) to find how many women would be married at that rate before the next birthday; those "casualties" are entered in the column M_x. With a completed N_x column we finally can derive, usually by interpolation, the column of most interest to us, the S_x column. S_x tells us the woman-years spent single between birthday x and birthday $x + 1$ by

[d]These are examples of gross nuptiality tables vs. net nuptiality tables. Net nuptiality tables express attrition from the single population both by means of first marriage and death operating concurrently. Gross nuptiality tables express attrition via marriage alone among those members of the cohort who survive mortality.

[e]Nuptiality tables have not yet become so conventionalized that all contain the same columns or even the same headings for similar columns. We present the terminology employed by the source, Donald Bogue, and also by Walter Mertens, who worked with Bogue in preparing the tables. We have left out five columns from the source tables irrelevant for our present purposes. Donald J. Bogue, *Principles of Demography* (New York: John Wiley & Sons, Inc., 1969), Tables 17-2 and 17-4.

[f]The estimation of *nuptiality* rates (as distinct from *marriage* rates) usually is the most difficult step in constructing a nuptiality table, just as the estimation of mortality rates (as distinct from death rates) is the most difficult in constructing a life table. The original source can be vital registration data and/or census data. See Mertens, "Construction of Nuptiality Tables."

the hypothetical cohort. It is very similar in meaning to the proportion of women single by age category for the hypothetical cohort of women such as those presented in Table 6-1 and Figure 6-1.

Figure 6-2 traces the n_x and S_x column for each of the two populations to illustrate the relationships between nuptiality rate schedule differences and differences in cohort single-status histories. The main point to be made from Figure 6-2 is that the relationship

Table 6-2

Abbreviated Nuptiality Tables for White and for Nonwhite Females, United States: 1950-1960

Age	White				Nonwhite			
	n_x	N_x	M_x	S_x	n_x	N_x	M_x	S_x
15	.0280	100000	2800	98600	.0400	100000	400	99800
16	.0500	97200	4860	94770	.0580	99600	5777	96712
17	.1000	92340	9234	87723	.0975	93823	9148	89249
18	.1750	83106	14544	75834	.1560	84675	13209	78070
19	.2130	68562	14604	61260	.1820	71466	13007	64962
20	.2370	53958	12788	47564	.1760	58459	10289	53314
21	.2500	41170	10293	36024	.1700	48170	8189	44075
22	.2580	30877	7966	26894	.1610	39981	6437	36762
23	.2275	22911	5212	20305	.1520	33544	5099	30995
24	.2000	17699	3540	15929	.1400	28445	3982	26454
25	.1775	14159	2513	12902	.1300	24463	3180	22873
26	.1550	11646	1805	10743	.1175	21283	2501	20032
27	.1370	9841	1348	9167	.1075	18782	2019	17772
28	.1200	8493	1019	7984	.0960	16763	1609	15958
29	.1070	7474	800	7074	.0855	15154	1296	14506
30	.0950	6674	634	6357	.0775	13858	1074	13321
31	.0840	6040	507	5786	.0680	12784	869	12350
32	.0745	5533	412	5327	.0600	11915	715	11558
33	.0655	5121	335	4954	.0525	11200	588	10906
34	.0575	4786	275	4648	.0460	10612	488	10368
35	.0500	4511	226	4398	.0400	10124	405	9922
36	.0455	4285	195	4188	.0350	9719	340	9549
37	.0410	4090	168	4006	.0310	9379	291	9233
38	.0375	3922	147	3849	.0260	9088	236	8970
39	.0350	3775	132	3709	.0225	8852	199	8752

Table 6-2 (cont.)

Age	White				Nonwhite			
	n_x	N_x	M_x	S_x	n_x	N_x	M_x	S_x
40	.0310	3643	113	3587	.0190	8653	164	8571
41	.0290	3530	102	3479	.0155	8489	132	8423
42	.0260	3428	89	3384	.0125	8357	104	8305
43	.0245	3339	82	3298	.0110	8253	91	8208
44	.0225	3257	73	3220	.0085	8162	69	8128
45	.0210	3184	67	3150	.0075	8093	61	8062
46	.0195	3117	61	3087	.0060	8032	48	8008
47	.0180	3056	55	3028	.0050	7984	40	7964
48	.0170	3001	51	2975	.0045	7944	36	7926
49	.0160	2950	47	2926	.0035	7908	28	7894
50	.0150	2903	44	2881	.0030	7880	24	7868

n_x = Nuptiality rate.
N_x = Never-married (single) at age x.
M_x = Number marrying at age x.
S_x = Person-years in never-married (single) status in year of x to $x + 1$.
Source: Bogue, Table 17-2 and 17-4 (see footnote e).

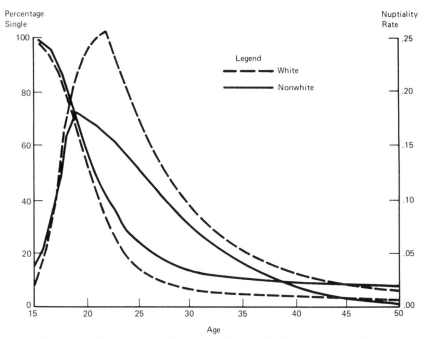

Figure 6-2. Percentages Single and Nuptiality Rates, by Age, White and Nonwhite Females, United States, 1950-1960. Source: table 6-2.

between nuptiality rate schedules and cohort single-status histories is complex. Compared with the white nuptiality rates, the nonwhite nuptiality rates peak earlier but are lower for every given year of age except the earliest teens. The net result of these two rate-schedule differences is to cause the nonwhites to have lower proportions single at every age starting with the late teens.

It seems likely that these two differences (earlier peaking and lower general age-specific rates) operated in different directions rather than in concert upon the proportions single. As preliminary generalizations, one might suppose that:

1. All else being equal, the earlier the peak nuptiality rate is reached, the lower the proportion single at later ages. The earlier peak will have eliminated more single women because the rate will have operated on a large number of single women.
2. All else being equal, the higher the nuptiality rates at given ages, the lower the proportions single at all later ages.

According to principle 1, the nonwhites should have had lower proportions single at later ages. According to principle 2, the nonwhites should have had higher proportions single at later ages. Apparently, the force of principle 2 was greater than that of principle 1.

This example emphasizes that we need more formal demographic work specifying the relationships between nuptiality schedules and cohort single status.[g] Nevertheless, our introduction to nuptiality tables should have alerted us to the fact that the first-marriage process has several aspects worth keeping separate conceptually. Let us elaborate further.

Important Dimensions of the First-Marriage Process

Because the first-marriage process can have such an impact upon period fertility, first marriage is likely to be the first focus of any

[g] A profitable starting place for such nuptiality study may be the adaptation of generalizations found in mortality study. See, for instance, Ansley J. Coale, "Birth Rates, Death Rates, and Rates of Growth in Human Population," in Mindel Sheps and Jean Claire Ridley, eds., *Public Health and Population Change: Current Research Issues* (Pittsburgh: University of Pittsburgh Press, 1965), pp. 245-65.

policy for reducing fertility by altering marital patterns. In that consideration, policymakers will need all the knowledge they can get about the social and demographic determinants of the first-marriage process.

A preliminary step in developing such a body of knowledge is identification of the dependent variables; that is, identifying the important dimensions of the first-marriage process for study. That is the purpose of this section.

One main criterion by which we should judge whether or not an aspect of the marriage process is important is whether it covaries with cohort single status from society to society. Coale recently has found an important uniformity in the first-marriage process, that is, a dimension on which societies apparently do not vary. This discovery allows us better to identify the remaining dimensions on which societies do vary.[3] Let us summarize.

The uniformity Coale found was in the female age pattern of the first-marriage process. Finding an empirical regularity in the age pattern of a demographic process is not unusual. We are used to the idea of mortality having a standard age pattern, irrespective of the general mortality levels: mortality risk is relatively high in infancy, low in youth and early adulthood, and then increases again to a high level at advanced ages. We already have noted a regular, though perhaps less uniform, pattern of fertility with female ages, irrespective of general fertility level: fertility is relatively low during the female teens, highest during the twenties, declining through the thirties, and approaching zero in the forties.[4]

Coale found a similar kind of empirical regularity regarding the proportions remaining single by female age and, by the same token, in the incidence of first marriage by female age. The basic form of the curves he identified is illustrated by our Figure 6-2, the percentage-single curves and the nuptiality-rate curves.

He first noticed the similarity among the European countries whose demographic transitions he was studying. Then, having identified the pattern, he brought in evidence from other regions and other times to assess its generality. He concludes:

The most puzzling feature of the common pattern of first-marriage frequencies is its very prevalence. We have seen evidence of the same basic curve of first marriage in cohorts that marry early and cohorts that marry late, in cohorts in which marriage is virtually universal, and in cohorts in which one-quarter remain single. Moreover, the uniform age structure of nuptiality occurs in societies in which most marriages are arranged by families with little regard for the preference of the bride and groom, and in societies in which marriages typically result from the self-selection of mutually preferred partners.[5]

Accordingly, Coale was able to propose a mathematical formula describing a standard schedule of the risk of first marriage by age. What is important for our purpose is what are the variables in the formula, that is, what is not uniform in the first-marriage processes of societies. Another quote from Coale pinpoints those important dimensions of variation.

The risk of first marriage in any cohort can be summarized as follows: (1) There is a convention that effectively prevents first marriage in the cohort before a minimum age defined by law, religion, or custom. (2) A fraction of the cohort is not in the marriage pool, because of such forces as the relative numbers of men and women whom members of the cohort marry, restrictions on marriage, including the provision of dowry, and traditions of celibacy. (3) The portion of the cohort in the marriage pool experiences a risk of marriage that rises from zero at the conventionally defined minimum age to a maximum risk that is maintained until the last marriages that occur to the cohort. . . .[6]

These, then, are the important dimensions of intersocietal variation with respect to the first-marriage process: (1) the female age at which the first-marriage process conventionally starts, (2) the proportion of the female population who never will marry, (3) the speed with which the first marriage process spreads through those females who ever are to marry.

It is these three factors that are the immediate determinants of cohort single status. Accordingly, any investigation of the social and demographic determinants of cohort single status via the first-marriage process should focus on these three factors as dependent variables. That, at least, is my advice to myself for the future.

Summary

The process of marriage continuously depletes single women from a cohort so that there are naturally a higher proportion of single women at younger reproductive ages than at older reproductive ages.

The younger ages characterized by relatively high proportions single normally include the early twenties, years particularly important in determining period fertility. During the early twenties, the woman-years spent outside of married status because of lack of first marriage is consistently more than the woman-years spent outside of married status because of widowhood and divorce combined. In Western countries, the proportion of women aged 20-24 still single is sizable.

The process of first marriage bears a close resemblance to the process of mortality. Accordingly, the nature of relationships between nuptiality and cohort single status can be described by borrowing a sophisticated model from mortality analysis, the life table, and constructing analogous nuptiality tables. Although nuptiality tables can be used to describe precisely the implications of assumed age schedules of nuptiality rates for cohort single status, we still lack generalizations about the relationships between these two variables.

Coale has found that the female age pattern of relative risk of first marriage varies little among societies. Rather, the first marriage process seems to vary with respect to: (1) the female age at which the first-marriage process normally starts, (2) the proportion of the female population who never will marry, and (3) the speed with which the first-marriage process spreads through those females who ever are to marry. These three variables, then, are advised as dependent variables for any study of the social and demographic determinants of the first-marriage process.

7

Implications for a Fertility-Reduction Policy

The immediate policy goal assumed in this chapter is cohort completed fertility low enough, and age at childbearing late enough, to attain zero national annual rates of natural increase in the presence of continued low mortality. In the initial chapter section we relate that goal to the end of global zero population growth.

The only means we consider are changing the incidence and pace of marital events. First we treat the only events which could be altered in order to influence cohort marital status: remarriage, divorce and widowhood, and first marriage. Then we deal with the likely effects of altered cohort marital status on fertility, treating especially the complex relationship between a marriage-reduction policy and a birth-control policy.

An introductory disclaimer here may avoid high hopes on the part of the reader and subsequent disappointment. We are not in position to make any final evaluation of the alternative marriage policies considered. Even if we accepted that goal, we lack two bodies of knowledge necessary for such an evaluation.

First, we have not gathered evidence regarding the other effects of any marriage policy to be considered. For example, even if we should conclude that a policy of increased divorce might result in fertility reduction, we have made no attempt in previous chapters to assess the other effects of a prodivorce policy relative to other ends, such as decreasing discord between marital partners, increasing stability in socialization of children, and so forth.

An exception to this generalization is our attention to illegitimacy as a possible side effect of marital reduction policies. In that case, Chapter 4 has armed us with some thoughts.

Second, we have not yet attended the secondary effects of any marriage policy with respect to fertility reduction itself. For example, it is conceivable that increasing the proportion of women who are in the status of divorced, for example, by deterring incidence of remarriage, might cause a shortage of eligible women in the marriage market and thus decrease the normal age at which unmarried women are defined as normally eligible. Such a lowering of the average age at first marriage would tend to push fertility up, countering the effect of increased divorce.

Assumed Policy Ends

Let us assume that the end of policy is eventual universal national zero annual rates of natural increase. This would be the only condition under which global zero population growth would occur, unless one anticipates appreciable net migration among nations even under conditions of increasing general population density. We make the goal a national one since it seems realistic to think that the agencies considering any such policy would be national governments, not some international agency nor localities within nations.

Let us assume that zero national increase is to be achieved solely through altering fertility: that is, assume that the policy really is one aimed at the end of national fertility reduction. It is unlikely that a policy end of increasing general mortality or shortening life expectancy ever will be acceptable to national governments.

By implication from the above assumptions, the goal of policy would be national period fertility rates low enough to balance national period death rates, which in turn are at the low levels now anticipated with modern technology. As a ball park figure let us suppose that this translates in cohort terms, in the long run, to slightly more than two—and certainly less than three—live births per woman. The later the average age of women at childbearing, the higher the range the permissible completed family size could be.[1]

Decreasing the Proportion Married
by Decreasing Remarriage

The marital events whose incidence and timing policy could influence are (1) first marriage, (2) marital dissolution through divorce or death of husband, and (3) remarriage. If period fertility reduction be the ultimate goal, then the proximate goal would be altering cohort marital status so that among fecund-aged women, and especially among women in their early twenties, the proportion married would be reduced.[a] This favorable influence on cohort marital status might be achieved (1) by decreasing the proportion of women who ever marry or by delaying the age at first marriage among those who ever marry, (2) by increasing the proportion of fecund-aged women who ever experience divorce or death of husband, or (3) by decreasing the proportion of the divorced or widowed women who ever remarry, or by delaying the speed with which those women who ever remarry do remarry. Let us take up these paths of action, starting with marital dissolution and remarriage, then treating first marriage.

Chapter 5 concluded that the impact of widowhood and divorce on marital status of young women was small and likely to remain so. However, that estimate was based on the assumption that remarriage of widows and divorcees would continue at a high level or increase in incidence and that it would continue to happen generally and rapidly to *young* women. If remarriage patterns and trends are such that they negate the effects of husbands' death and divorce on female cohort marital status, then why not consider *policies for altering patterns of remarriage*?

Policies for influencing remarriage negatively might include (1) policies for reducing the proportion of widows and divorces ever remarrying or (2) policies for increasing the time between the event of husband's death or divorce and remarriage of the woman. Category (1) might include instituting remarriage eligibility requirements on various bases, including even maximum number of living children.[b] Category (2) might include stating a minimum female age for remarriage or a minimum time gap between divorce and/or widowhood and remarriage. There are, of course, ways other than direct governmental decrees for achieving both effects (1) and (2), such as through tax benefits.

If the tendency for higher divorce rates to accompany westernization continues, then also the potential impact of such a remarriage-reduction policy increases. Whereas widowhood is more likely to occur among older women, divorce does not follow such an automatic age pattern and happens to women in young and fecund ages as well.[2] Therefore, if there were no remarriage, the shift from widowhood to divorce as the reason for marital dissolution would

---

[a]Chapters 2 and 3.

[b]Such a policy would be particularly effective if selection for remarriage eligibility could be made on the basis of demonstrated low fecundity. Chapter 3.

result in a shift toward a younger average age of nonremarried woman.

Moreover, one could argue that the women being kept in the nonmarried status by such policies would be those least likely to suffer fertility outside of marriage. Whereas never-married women are presumably less experienced in contraception, married women are presumably more likely to have developed such skills while married. Remarriage reduction is likely to result in less increased illegitimacy than is first-marriage reduction, according to this argument.[c,d]

There are many ways in which remarriage could be discouraged or delayed. One possibility would be to facilitate legal separation but to hinder divorce, with its implication of permission for remarriage. Another possibility would be to provide generous economic welfare benefits for widowed and divorced women so they would be less driven to remarriage in order to survive financially and to provide for their children. Another would be to increase the occupational alternatives open to women so that divorced and widowed women would not be driven to a new wife-mother position for lack of choices.

Decreasing the Proportion Married
by Increasing Widowhood and Divorce

The proportion of young women in the status of widowed is determined by the events of husband's death and of widow's remarriage. Holding prospects for remarriage constant for the moment, how might the incidence of husband's death be influenced in order to maximize the proportion of young women who are widows? The tactic of increasing general mortality would seldom be

---

[c]On the other hand, it is possible that any policy discouraging remarriage also will discourage divorce. To the degree that anticipation of certain and rapid remarriage was a factor in the marital dissolution, then this would be the case. Determining the truth of that assertion, however, is beyond the scope of this book.

[d]Another possible side effect of any remarriage-reduction policy would be to take formerly eligible women out of the marriage market and thus possibly to increase the demand for the remaining women, and this might in turn drive down the average age of women at first marriage. Whether such assumptions about the effect of partner shortage on age at marriage are valid is problematical and beyond the scope of this book. However, even if the theory were valid, the hypothesized effect rests on the assumption that only women were taken out of the marriage pool. It could be obviated by forbidding or delaying the remarriage of widowed and divorced men as well.

a permissible policy. However, there are ways in which the mortality pattern might be influenced so that an indirect effect would be to maximize the proportion of women who were widowed. Greater emphasis could be placed on reducing female mortality than male mortality within the context of a general mortality-reduction policy.[e] Any tendency for widows to have higher age-specific mortality than married women could be counteracted. The age gap at marriage could be influenced so that the husband normally was increasingly older than the wife, and thus would suffer increasingly higher relative risk of death. And, to be complete, women could be encouraged to marry at earlier ages so that they would experience the risk of husband's death for longer periods, although any such policy would also probably increase the proportion of young women who were ever married.

Under conditions of low probability of remarriage or long delay of remarriage, a policy of encouraging divorce, and especially young divorce could have an appreciable effect on cohort marital status. Divorce tends to replace widowhood as a means of marital dissolution with modernization and the decline in general mortality, and therefore influencing the divorce rate upward would have an increasing potential impact. Moreover, the age at which divorce normally occurs is spread rather evenly through the female ages rather than being aggregated in the later ages, as is the case with widowhood.

A variety of policies for encouraging divorce come to mind. One method would be to increase the grounds admissable for divorce. Another method would be to make the life of divorced women more tolerable to contemplate, by offering welfare and occupational roles, as suggested above under discouraging remarriage. However, one method likely to encourage divorce, but obviously fruitless in increasing the proportion of women staying in divorced status, would be to make remarriage likely and rapid.

The ways for making divorces earlier rather than later in the lives of women are less obvious. One possibility would be to make divorce or separation especially easy for those with no children or few children.[f]

---

[e]As a secondary effect, this would create a shortage of men in the marriage market, thus perhaps increasing the proportion of women who never married, or never remarried.

[f]Such a policy might be counterproductive in that high-fecundity women might be selected for continuation of marriage while subfecund women might have greater likelihood of divorce.

Decreasing the Proportion Married by Decreasing and Delaying First Marriage

The first-marriage process remains the avenue by which cohort marital status is most vulnerable to change in a manner which ultimately will reduce fertility. This is true even if the remarriage and marital dissolution patterns can be altered as suggested above. If remarriage cannot be avoided or deferred, then first marriage is the only avenue remaining for altering cohort marital status.

The three aspects of the first-marriage process susceptible to influence are the proportion of women ever marrying, the age at which first marriage normally starts, and the speed with which it proceeds after starting. We conclude from Coale's work that these aspects are distinct enough for policymakers to consider affecting them separately.[3]

How promising is reduction of the proportion of women ever marrying? On the one hand, it suffers from diffusion of its impact, since it does not focus its effect on women in their twenties. On the other hand, it compares favorably with marital dissolution as an avenue in that it at least does not focus its impact on the less fecund later ages as they tend to.

Relatively speaking, however, the path of influencing age at first marriage is far the more promising. By the very nature of the process, increased age at first marriage increases nonmarried status in the early female years, including the crucial highly fecund ages of the twenties.

Average female age at first marriage is a factor of two aspects of the first-marriage process identified by Coale, the normal age at which first marriage proceeds and the speed with which it then proceeds through the population of women who ever are to be married.[4] Both of these aspects of the process could be viewed as paths by which average age at first marriage could be altered.

I am not prepared at this point to suggest means by which either the proportion ever marrying can be reduced or by which the initiation and pace of first marriage be detained. Such suggestions rest upon a theoretical formulation of the demographic and non-demographic determinants of the first-marriage process. Although promising beginnings have been made in developing the needed theory, it seems not yet ready for succinct summary in this context. I regard the development of such theory as of highest scientific priority in the study of policies for fertility reduction.

Decreasing Proportions Married and Fertility: A Classification of Situations

Up to this point we have been treating the ways in which marital events could be altered in order to change cohort marital status. Those thoughts have value only to the degree that such changes in cohort marital status can contribute to fertility reduction. At this point we address ourselves to the following question: Under what conditions is a reduction of the proportion of women in their twenties who are married most likely to result in a reduction of fertility?

To put order in that consideration, it is helpful to consider a simple typology, presented in Figure 7-1. The typology distinguishes four sets of conditions in which nations might find themselves at the time they contemplate a policy of reducing the proportion of young women who are married. Only two dimensions of variation are recognized, though undoubtedly a more sophisticated typology could helpfully include more.

One dimension is *ability* in birth control. Included in that dimension is degree of social acceptability of, and individual skill in, contraception and/or induced abortion. Being high on this dimension, however, does not necessarily mean employing that capacity in order to achieve low fertility.

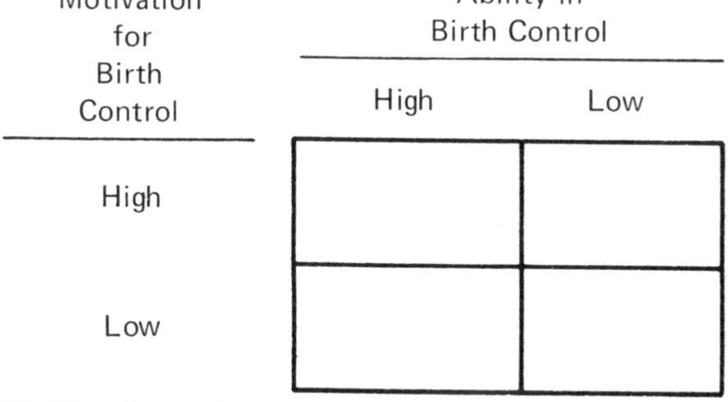

Motivation for Birth Control	Ability in Birth Control	
	High	Low
High		
Low		

Figure 7-1. Typology of National Conditions Based on Ability in, and Motivation for, Birth Control.

The other dimension is the *motivation* to limit fertility. A high motivation to limit fertility would be provided by a desire for a small family, a desire to space children, *or a desire to avoid bearing children in a socially unacceptable status such as nonmarried.*

It is our contention that cohort marital status influences fertility primarily by increasing the *motivation* to limit fertility. Since, by definition, all societies have sanctions against illegitimate birth, individuals and groups within the society universally tend to avoid those negative sanctions by adjusting behavior with respect to the Davis-Blake intermediate variables. For instance, families to which the potential partners belong tend to isolate them from sexual contact prior to marriage. Or the potential partners themselves tend to limit sexual contact or to guard against conception or birth as a result. Thus nonmarried status furnishes potential partners with additional motivation to avoid birth, to use birth control.

Each of the two dimensions is dichotomized, then the two dimensions are cross-classified to produce four types: high-motivation/high-ability; high-motivation/low-ability; low-motivation/high-ability; low-motivation/low-ability. Into the high-motivation/high-ability class would fall most of the "post-transitional" countries of European culture. Into the low-motivation/low-ability class would fall most presently underdeveloped countries, relatively speaking.

Decreasing Proportions Married
Under Conditions of High Motivation
and High Ability for Birth Control

Let us first treat the situation where there is both a high level of motivation for reducing fertility in the country and also a high general level of ability for reducing fertility. We first encountered this situation of high-motivation/high-ability in Chapter 3, and have some more detailed thoughts on record there.

The general point was and is that under conditions of high motivation and high ability most of the impact of a reduction in marriage upon fertility would be obviated. Under the conditions that all women had a small desired family size (say three children) and all were ever married, then a delay in the age at first marriage or a prolongation of periods of marital interruption could easily be overcome voluntarily by the woman. In a sense, under these conditions a policy to increase motivation for control by bringing to bear the sanctions against illegitimacy would be redundant: the women already are motivated.

However, some qualifications are appropriate. First, suppose the pattern of marriage reduction was such that it increased the proportion of women who never married rather than simply delaying the average age at which women married or shortening periods of marital interruption. Then the women who never married would be motivated to have no children rather than the assumed three they would have sought had they married. Aggregate motivation for control would have been increased.

A second qualification deals with the influence of cohort marital status on the timing of births. If we suppose that the thrust of the marriage-control policy was to reduce the proportion of women aged 20-29 who were married without necessarily reducing the proportion of women of later ages who were married to the same degree, then one effect would be to increase the average age at childbearing. This, in turn, would have a minor negative effect on period fertility even if all women ended up with the assumed three children.[5]

In sum, under conditions of high motivation and high ability for fertility reduction, marital reduction is likely to have little impact upon the completed family size of those women who eventually do marry. However, it still could reduce aggregate fertility by increasing the proportion of women who never do marry and thus the proportion who want never to have any children and also by increasing the age of childbearing for those women who do marry.[6]

Decreasing the Proportion Married
Under Conditions of High Motivation
and Low Ability for Birth Control

The impact of decreased female proportions married during the ages 20-29 would seem to reach its nadir under conditions of existing high motivation and low ability for birth control. This follows from our premise that nonmarriage influences fertility primarily through increasing motivation to avoid birth. There already is a surfeit of such motivation under the conditions we are assuming.

Indeed, increasing the proportion of young women nonmarried under these circumstances is likely to have dominantly a negative side effect: the proportions of births which are illegitimate is likely to increase. Unwanted births which otherwise at least would have occurred within marriage now would occur outside of marriage.

Decreasing the Proportion Married
Under Conditions of Low Motivation
and High Ability for Birth Control

The situation in which a marriage reduction policy is likely to have maximal impact is the situation in which there exists a low motivation for fertility reduction but a high ability to achieve any such desired reduction through voluntary birth control. The reason for this is simply that marriage reduction operates primarily through altering motivation for control, and motivation for control here is all that is lacking. Unmarried, divorced, or widowed women would, under these conditions, be able to avoid conception and birth.

A second point to be made is that these conditions are exceedingly rare, on a national level, and certainly do not exist in the countries of most rapid population growth. The closest approximation to the described situation might be the "marriage boom" and "baby boom" immediately after World War II in Europe and the United States.

To the degree that national family-planning programs in countries of rapid population growth do succeed, however, they will be bringing those countries closer to a situation in which marital reduction policies can add their contribution. This is the reason for our conclusion, in Chapter 4, that family planning and marital reduction policies should not be conceived as alternatives but rather as mutually dependent.

Decreasing Proportions Married Under
Conditions of Low Motivation and Low
Ability for Birth Control

Almost all countries of rapid population growth today fall within this type. And it is for this type that marital reduction as a policy is most frequently suggested.

To the degree that ability to employ birth control is absent, then the effect of increasing motivation for control by reducing the proportion of young women who are married depends on the presence of other means for limiting fertility. If there are means for avoiding intercourse during women's youth, then nonmarriage still can reduce fertility via that path. But the general trends of change in family institutions, as summarized by Goode, certainly do not indicate a persistence or growth in the capacity of extended families to shelter their women; quite the contrary. One can imagine other means of social control, such as isolation of sexes in communes, being employed, but they are so unlikely to be acceptable on a worldwide scale that we will not treat them seriously here.

A marital reduction unaccompanied by fertility reduction would have the universally undesired consequence of higher illegitimacy. This already has been illustrated historically in the case of Europe during the 1800s in Chapter 4. This prospect alone is likely to make a policy of marital reduction frightening to countries in which birth control ability is not yet general or imminent.

The conclusion is not that a marital reduction policy would not serve to limit fertility in countries of existing low motivation and low ability for birth control. Rather the conclusion is that the increased motivation for birth control potentially supplied by marital reduction must have some means to be implemented, or illegitimacy will result. That means for implementation could be supplied by an intense family-planning program simultaneous to, or prior to, any marital reduction.

It is important to note, however, that a conventional family planning would not work well. The people whose skills at birth control need improving are the nonmarried women. Conventional family-planning programs aim at married couples and indeed sometimes take great pains to deny that they increase skill and use among the nonmarried. The paradox is that few nations are likely to pursue policies of birth control for nonmarrieds since that usually will be seen as a policy of encouraging sexual immorality. It is a moot question how quickly a family-planning program aimed at the general population would reach the unmarried.

Tentative Conclusions

1. The focus of any marriage-reduction policy aimed at the goal of period-fertility reduction should be increasing the proportion of

women in their twenties, and especially their early twenties, who are nonmarried.

2. Such a marriage-reduction policy is likely to have minimal effect on fertility where individual ability in voluntary birth control is low. It might be effective in technologically developed countries, though it is likely to be redundant there. In technologically underdeveloped countries, any policy for marriage reduction should be preceded by or accompanied by a policy for increasing skill in voluntary birth control, especially among the nonmarried.

3. A marriage-reduction policy is a plausible adjunct for a fertility-reduction policy in technologically underdeveloped countries. Reducing the proportion of young women who are married can increase the motivation to use the voluntary birth control measures being introduced.

4. One means of marriage reduction worth attention is that of reducing remarriage, possibly, but not necessarily, in combination with selectively facilitating divorce and separation.

5. The main thrust of any marriage-reduction policy should be reducing and/or delaying first marriage. In technologically developed countries, the impact of a delay in age at marriage would be minimal and should be supplemented by a strong component to reduce proportions of women ever marrying. In technologically underdeveloped countries, in contrast, the initial focus should still be on delay of first marriage.

6. Any national policy including marriage reduction and family planning will have to accommodate itself to the likelihood that it is increasing the proportion of sexual encounters that take place outside of marriage. One policy goal, therefore, should be to reinforce social sanctions against birth outside marriage while not reinforcing social sanctions against contraception and abortion used outside marriage. Sanctions should be focused on reproduction, not sex.

Some Speculation about the Prospects

This is the final section of a very taut chapter of a fairly taut book. Let me now indulge myself in some loose speculation.

Let us first review what policy means have been suggested in the chapter. Then let us try to assess reasons for optimism or pessimism about these means being socially acceptable to national governments. I will start with a statement of the most pessimistic view, and then try to find rays of hope.[7]

First, a review of the proposed strategy: One element would be to encourage the capacity of unmarried women to avoid giving birth, either by supplying constraints against intercourse or, more likely, by increasing unmarried couples' ability at voluntary contraception or abortion. Given this capacity for holding illegitimate fertility at a low level, the other elements of the strategy would consist of various means of reducing the proportion of women who were married during parts of their reproductive years, and especially in their twenties. One path might be by increasing the incidence of marital dissolution through death of husband or divorce. But the dominant path would be through reduction of marriage, whether it be through the delay or reduction of remarriage of widows or divorcees or—potentially more important—through the delay and reduction of first marriage.

A conventional functionalist view of societal organization leads one to be rather pessimistic about such policy means being implemented broadly. Let me state the view in fairly simplistic terms: Historically, all societies have lived with persistent high mortality until the very recent past. Therefore, cultural patterns and values developed which universally resulted in high fertility to overcome the high mortality and avert the eventual disappearance of the society. Aspects of the culture associated with this vital reproductive process are particularly basic in the culture because of their importance, and therefore they are particularly resistant to change. Key among these cultural patterns related to fertility are those surrounding the institution which, by definition, is centrally involved in legitimate reproduction: the family. Consequently, changing family patterns which support high fertility is likely to be especially difficult.

Let us avoid, for the moment, a debate about the virtues of functionalism as a sociological frame of reference. Instead, let us try to see any departures from the general picture presented above that improve our expectation of fertility reduction via marriage reduction.

First, it is erroneous to suppose that the cultural forms surrounding the family always resulted in unrestricted fertility. Indeed, one could say that the family as an institution itself represents a restriction on fertility. By defining some units, marriages, as uniquely appropriate for reproduction, all other units are by implication defined as inappropriate, and reproduction in other unions is defined as illegitimate. Nor is there anything new about societies setting up elaborate procedures for cutting down the incidence of illegitimate fertility.

If one takes this view, then, the prospects for social acceptance of additional controls over illegitimacy seem less bleak. Moreover, if growing illegitimacy should be defined as a social problem, it seems likely that societies would be willing to overcome some existing qualms about techniques in order to solve such a potentially disorganizing problem. Thus I would not be surprised to see societies openly facilitating use of contraception and induced abortion among nonmarried couples if high illegitimacy rates threatened.

Second, any such tidy description of a culture as the one above is likely to result in a stereotypical view of the values actually held in the population. Foreign sociologists, and even native national leaders, have been fooled before by the disparity between the cultural ideal and the real. An example was the general belief that the traditional cultures of technologically underdeveloped countries involved a valuation of high and unlimited fertility by married couples. National leaders and sociologists were quite adept at giving functional reasons for such high-fertility desires. But when the facts came in, with the international wave of fertility surveys in the 1960s, what evidence they produced supported the view that moderate fertility was the general desire, not high and unlimited fertility; for example, three or four children vs. the six or seven children that couples were having on the average.

Is it possible that we are misleading ourselves also about the values held regarding marriage practices in contemporary societies? Do people really abhor an increased probability of divorce or is serial polygamy an enticing prospect? Is early marriage really every maiden's dream, or only early sex without shame? Does every divorcee really want to try again as soon as possible, or are there simply few options offered?

Third, any specific proposed change is likely to relate to not only those cultural values surrounding the family system, but other values as well. In some cases these other values will be against the proposed change, but in other cases they may support it and overcome any inherent conservatism of the family system.

An illustration of the first kind of outcome is the case of increased widowhood. Even if increasing husband mortality were not defined as a threat to the family institution, the generalized high valuation of longevity probably would militate against any policy with mortality increase as a stated goal.

On the other hand, some of the specific steps one might conceive for reducing the incidence of marriage and remarriage might be in accord with other values and gain support from that accord. Tax discrimination against unmarried men and women can be abhorred on the basis of the principle of fair play. Offering better occupational opportunities to women can be argued for on the basis of egalitarian ideology. Permission of induced abortion to unmarried women can be argued for on the basis of increased individual freedom.

Fourth, it is misleading to view cultures as static, at least in the major nations of the contemporary world. Changes are taking place, and particularly changes are taking place in family systems. Moreover, the direction of the change associated with modernization on the Western model is generally change in the direction of marriage reduction: First marriage tends to get later. Larger proportions of women never marry. Divorce increases in incidence. Thus, while the proposed policy means may be inconsistent with the simplified picture of a traditional society, they seem quite consistent with the general drift of changes as those societies modernize.

Nevertheless, the dispute between the optimistic and pessimistic views cannot be resolved at this time because too many facts have yet to come in. We probably can agree that the key policies will be those influencing the incidence of marriage and remarriage. (That is, it is unlikely that an increase in the incidence of either husbands' death or divorce will be the central thrust of any marriage-reduction policy.) But we have just begun to explore what might be done to reduce and delay marriage. It might be something as direct as passing a law demanding that women be a certain minimum age at marriage. On the other hand, it might be something as devious as encouraging sex-selective internal migration in order to create imbalances in local marriage markets. Until we have a clearer idea about the determinants of the female first-marriage process, and thus the factors which can be manipulated in order to influence it, pessimism about the social acceptability of policies seems premature at least.

Notes

Notes

Chapter 1
Introduction

1. Kingsley Davis, "Population Policy: Will Current Programs Succeed?" *Science* 158 (November 10, 1967): 730-39; also see the exchange of letters in later issues of that journal. Judith Blake, "Population Policy for Americans: Is the Government Being Misled?" *Science* 164 (May 2, 1969): 522-29; also see the exchange of letters in subsequent issues. Judith Blake, "Reproductive Motivation and Population Policy," *BioScience* 21 (March 1, 1971): 215-20. Frank W. Notestein, "Zero Population Growth," *Population Index* 36 (October-December, 1970): 444-52; also see the comments by Philip M. Hauser, Judith Blake, and Paul Demeny recorded on pages 452-65 of that journal. Bernard Berelson, "Beyond Family Planning," *Studies in Family Planning* 38 (February 1969): 1-16.

2. Davis, "Population Policy," p. 737.

3. See Chapter 7.

4. Malini Karkal, *Annotated Bibliography of Studies on Age at Marriage in India* (Bombay: International Institute of Population Studies, 1971). S N Agarwala *Age at Marriage in India* (Allahabad: Kitab Mahal, Ltd., 1962). Murari Majumdar and Ajit Das Gupta, "Marriage Trends and Their Demographic Implications," *Sankya* (Calcutta), ser. B 31 (3-4) (December 1969): 491-500.

5. Note 1, above.

6. Ansley J. Coale, "The Decline of Fertility in Europe from the French Revolution to World War II," in S.J. Behrman, L. Corsa, and R. Freedman (eds.), *Fertility and Family Planning: A World View* (Ann Arbor: University of Michigan Press, 1969), pp. 3-25. Norman B. Ryder, "The Character of Modern Fertility," *The Annals of the American Academy of Political and Social Science,* (January 1967): 26-36. These scholars express their debt to the pioneering work of John Hajnal such as in his "European Marriage Patterns in Perspective," in D.V. Glass and D.E.C. Eversley (eds.), *Population in History: Essays in Historical Demography* (London: Edward Arnold, Ltd., 1965), pp. 100-143.

7. David Yaukey, "On Theorizing About Fertility," *American Sociologist*, 4 (May 1969): 100-104.

8. Kingsley Davis and Judith Blake, "Social Structure and Fertility: An Analytical Framework," *Economic Development and Cultural Change*, 4 (April 1956): 211-35. Ronald Freedman, "Applications of the Behavioral Sciences to Family Planning Programs," *Studies in Family Planning*, 23 (October 1967): 5-9.

Chapter 2
Period Fertility and Cohort Fertility

1. Chapter 1, note 4, above.

2. Norman B. Ryder, "The Process of Demographic Translation," *Demography* 1 (1964): 74-82.

3. A major theme of the Presidents Commission of Population and American Future has been the momentum toward high period fertility in the United States for the next several decades resulting from the abnormally large size of the baby boom female cohorts. See *Population and the American Future* (Washington: Superintendent of Documents, U.S. Government Printing Office, 1972). The combined influence of a variety of cohort fertility assumptions and projected U.S. female cohort sizes are spelled out by Thomas Frejka, "Reflections on the Demographic Conditions Needed to Establish a U.S. Stationary Population Growth," *Population Studies*, 22 (November 1968): 379-97.

4. Ansley J. Coale and C.Y. Tye, "The Significance of Age Patterns of Fertility in Highly Fertile Populations," *Milbank Memorial Fund Quarterly*, 29 (October 1961): 632-46.

5. Ibid., p. 643.

Chapter 3
Cohort Fertility and Marital Status

1. Kingsley Davis and Judith Blake, "Social Structure and Fertility: An Analytic Framework," *Economic Development and Cultural Change* 6 (April 1956): 211-35.

2. Ibid., p. 211.

3. Ibid., p. 212 (fn. 2) and pp. 214-15.

4. M.J. Bourgeois-Pichat, "Les Facteurs de la Fecondite Non Dirigee," *Population* 20 (1965): 383-424.

5. Geoffrey Hawthorne, *Sociology of Fertility* (London: Collier-MacMillan Ltd., 1970), p. 21. Hajnal, "European Marriage Patterns."

6. Ansley J. Coale, "Factors Associated with the Development of Low Fertility: An Historic Summary," in United Nations Department of Economic and Social Affairs, *World Population Conference, 1965*, II, (New York: United Nations, 1967), Table 1, p. 209.

7. Louis Henry, "French Statistical Research in Natural Fertility," in Mindel C. Sheps and Jeanne Clare Ridley (eds.) *Public Health and Population Change: Current Research Issues* (Pittsburgh: University of Pittsburgh Press, 1965), pp. 346-47.

8. Anrudh Kumar Jain, "Fecundability in Relation to Age in Taiwanese Women," *Population Studies* 23 (March 1969): 79-80.

9. Louis Henry, "Research in Natural Fertility," pp. 347-48.

10. Larry Bumpass, "Age at Marriage as a Variable in Socio-Economic Differentials in Fertility," *Demography* 6 (1) (February 1969): 52-53.

11. Edwin D. Driver, *Differential Fertility in Central India* (Princeton: Princeton University Press, 1963), pp. 78-80.

Chapter 4
Fertility of the Nonmarried

1. For examples of estimates employing the assumption of no illegitimate fertility see (chronologically listed) David Yaukey, *Fertility Differences in a Modernizing Country: A Survey of Lebanese Couples* (Princeton: Princeton University Press, 1961), pp. 52-53; J. William Leasure, "Malthus, Marriage and Multiplication," *Milbank Memorial Fund Quarterly* 41 (October 1963) I: 419-35; Ansley J. Coale, "The Decline of Fertility in Europe from the French Revolution to World War II," in S.J. Behrman, L. Corsa, and R. Freedman (eds.), *Fertility and Family Planning: A World View* (Ann Arbor: University of Michigan Press, 1969), pp. 3-25; Murari Majumdar and Ajit Das Gupta, "Marriage Trends and Their Demographic Implications," *Sankhya* (Calcutta) ser. B-31; (December 1969): 491-500; R. Lesthaeghe, "Nuptiality and Population Growth," *Population Studies* 25 (November 1971): 415-32.

2. Kingsley Davis, "Population Policy: Will Current Programs Succeed," *Science* 158 (November 10, 1967): 737.

3. Judith Blake, "Parental Control, Delayed Marriage, and Population Policy," *Proceedings of the World Population Conference, 1965* (New York: United Nations, 1967), 2, p. 132.

4. Norman B. Ryder, "The Character of Modern Fertility," *Annals of the American Academy of Political and Social Science* 369 (January 1967): 20.

5. Kingsley Davis and Judith Blake, "Social Structure and Fertility: An Analytical Framework," *Economic Development and Cultural Change*, 4 (April 1956): 212.

6. William Petersen, *Population*, (2nd ed.; London: Collier-MacMillan Ltd., 1969), p. 154.

7. Thomas R. Malthus, *An Essay on the Principle of Population* (2nd ed.; London, 1803) p. 512.

8. United Nations, *Demographic Yearbook, 1968, Special Topic: Marriage and Divorce Statistics* (New York: United Nations, 1969), Table 7.

9. Massimo Livi-Bacci, *A Century of Portuguese Fertility* (Princeton: Princeton University Press, 1971) pp. 53-54.

10. John Knodel, "Two and Half Centuries of Demographic History in a Bavarian Village," *Population Studies* 24 (November 1970): 366.

11. William Petersen, "The Demographic Transition in the Netherlands," *American Sociological Review* 25 (June 1960): 345.

12. E.A. Wrigley, *Population and History* (New York: McGraw-Hill, 1969), p. 88.

13. Edward Shorter, John Knodel, and Etienne Van De Walle, "The Decline of Non-Marital Fertility in Europe, 1880-1940," *Population Studies* 25 (November 1971): 383.

14. For a description of the changing relations between sexuality and illegitimacy during the eighteenth and nineteenth century in Europe, see Edward Shorter, "Illegitimacy, Sexual Revolution, and Social Change in Modern Europe," *Journal of Interdisciplinary History* 2 (Autumn 1971): 235-72.

15. These can be identified as publications since 1965 about Europe by Massimo Livi Bacci, Ansley J. Coale, Paul Demeny, John Knodel, Edward Shorter, and Etienne Van De Walle. Coale, in turn, gives due credit for complementary work, especially on earlier periods in Europe, by scholars from the (French) Institut National d'Etudes Demographiques and from the (English) Cambridge Group

for the History of Population and Social Structure. Coale, "Decline of Fertility in Europe," p. 10.

16. John Hajnal, "European Marriage Patterns in Perspective," in D.V. Glass and D.E.C. Eversley (eds.), *Population in History: Essays in Historical Demography* (London: Edward Arnold Ltd., 1965), p. 101.

17. Chapters 5 and 6 treat in greater detail the relation between marital events and marital status composition.

18. Hajnal, "European Marriage Patterns," p. 102, Table 2.

19. Shorter, Knodel, and Van de Walle, "Decline of Non-Marital Fertility in Europe," Figure I, p. 377. We have eliminated Shorter's lines for Greece, Hungary, and Bulgaria, since they fall outside our region of reference. We eliminated his data for 1950 and 1960 because they fall after our time of reference.

20. Ibid., p. 379. I am indebted to Van de Walle for pointing out that the summation sign in the denominator had been omitted in the article through a printing error.

21. Coale, "Decline of Fertility in Europe," map 2.

22. Joginder Kumar, "Demographic Analysis of Data on Illegitimate Births," *Social Biology* 16 (July 1969): Tables 7 and 14, pp. 100 and 105.

23. Livi-Bacci, *Portuguese Fertility* p. 60.

24. Massimo Livi Bacci, "Fertility and Population Growth in Spain in the Eighteenth and Nineteenth Centuries," *Daedalus* (Spring 1968): 530.

25. Shirley Hartley, "The Amazing Rise of Illegitimacy in Great Britain," *Social Forces* 44 (June 1966): 537.

26. Hajnal, "European Marriage Patterns," pp. 112-13.

27. Shorter, Knodel, and Van de Walle, "Decline of Non-Marital Fertility in Europe," pp. 376-77.

28. Coale, "Decline of Fertility in Europe," pp. 9-10.

29. Ansley J. Coale, "Factors Associated with the Development of Low Fertility: An Historic Summary," *Proceedings of the World Population Conference, 1965* (New York: United Nations, 1967), vol. II, pp. 205-209. Massimo Livi Bacci, "Fertility and Nuptiality Changes in Spain from the Late 18th Century to the Early 20th Century; Part Two," *Population Studies* 22 (July 1968): 200. Massimo Livi Bacci, *Portuguese Fertility*, p. 40.

30. Coale, "Decline of Fertility in Europe," Figure 3. p. 23.

Etienne Van de Walle, "Marriage and Marital Fertility," *Daedalus* 97 (Spring 1968), Figure 1, p. 492. Paul Demeny, "Early Fertility Decline in Austria-Hungary: A Lesson in the Demographic Transition," *Daedalus* 97 (Spring 1968): 516-17. John Knodel, "Law, Marriage, and Illegitimacy in Nineteenth Century Germany," *Population Studies* 20 (March 1967): 288.

31. Phillips Cutright, "Illegitimacy: Myths, Causes, and Cures," *Family Planning Perspectives* 3 (January 1971): 26.

32. Shorter, Knodel, and Van de Walle, "Decline of Non-Marital Fertility in Europe," p. 275.

33. Ryder, "Character of Modern Fertility," p. 31.

34. Kingsley Davis, "The Theory of Change and Response in Modern Demographic History," *Population Index* (October 1963), p. 345. Davis proceeds to cite evidence gathered by Glass regarding eight northwest European countries. D.V. Glass, *Population Policies and Movements in Europe* (Oxford: Clarendon Press, 1940), pp. 278-80.

35. Shorter, Knodel, and Van de Walle, "Decline of Non-Marital Fertility in Europe," pp. 380-83, 392.

36. Knodel, "Law, Marriage, and Illegitimacy," pp. 279-94. John Knodel, "Two and a Half Centuries of Demographic History in a Bavarian Village," *Population Studies* 24 (November 1970): 353-76.

37. Shorter, Knodel, and Van de Walle, "Decline of Non-Marital Fertility in Europe," p. 376.

38. Lesthaeghe, "Nuptiality and Population Growth," p. 426.

Chapter 5
Cohort Marital Status and
Marital Dissolution

1. Eduardo Arriaga, "The Effect of a Decline in Mortality on the Gross Reproduction Rate," *Milbank Memorial Fund Quarterly* 55 (July 1967): 334.

2. Bogue, *Demography*, p. 569.

3. Andrew Collver, "The Family Cycle in India and the United States," *American Sociological Review* 28 (February 1963): 94.

4. Kingsley Davis and Judith Blake, "Social Structure and Fertility: An Analytic Framework," *Economic Development and Cultural Change* 4 (April 1956): 227-28.

5. Kingsley Davis, *The Population of India and Pakistan* (Princeton: Princeton University Press, 1951), pp. 80-81.

6. It is questioned, for instance by Moni Nag, in *Factors Affecting Human Fertility in Nonindustrial Societies: A Cross-Cultural Study* (Yale University Publications in Anthropology, Number 66; New Haven, Conn.: Department of Anthropology, Yale University, 1962), pp. 101-102.

7. William J. Goode, *World Revolution and Family Patterns* (New York: The Free Press, 1963), pp. 10-26.

8. Bogue, *Demography* p. 647;

9. United Nations, *Demographic Yearbook*, 1968 (New York: United Nations, 1969), pp. 13-14.

10. Bogue, *Demography* p. 342.

11. Paul H. Jacobson, "Differentials in Divorce by Duration of Marriage and Size of Family," *American Sociological Review* 15 (April 1950): 235-244. William M. Kephart, "The Duration of Marriage," *American Sociological Review* 19 (June 1954): 209, cited by Gerard R. Leslie, *The Family in Social Context* (New York: Oxford University Press, 1967), pp. 597-598. Hugh Carter and Paul C. Glick, *Marriage and Divorce: A Social and Economic Study* (Cambridge, Mass.: Harvard University Press, 1970), Table 3-5. U.S. Department of Health, Education and Welfare, *Vital Statistics of the United States: 1960, Volume III, Marriage and Divorce*, Table 3E, cited in Bogue, *Demography*, p. 649.

12. Bogue, *Demography*, pp. 647-650.

13. Goode, *World Revolution*.

14. Ibid., pp. 155-162, 359-365, 195-198.

15. Ibid., pp. 81-86. Leslie, *Family in Social Context*, p. 586.

16. Carter and Glick, *Marriage and Divorce* Table 3-8, p. 54. Rate used was number of divorces per 1,000 married women aged fifteen years or more.

17. Ibid., p. 57. Abbot L. Ferriss, "An Indicator of Marriage Dissolution by Marriage Cohort," *Social Forces* 48 (March 1970): 364. U.S. Bureau of the Census, Current Population Reports, series P-20, no. 242, "Marital Status and Living Arrangements: March 1972," U.S. Government Printing Office, Washington, D.C., 1972, pp. 3-4.

18. Goode, *World Revolution* pp. 10-26.

19. Bernard Farber, *Family Organization and Interaction* (San Francisco: Chandler Publishing Co., 1964), pp. 104-111, 120.

20. Goode, *World Revolution*, p. 376; and William J. Goode, *After Divorce* (New York: The Free Press of Glencoe, 1956), p. 216.

21. Carter and Glick, *Marriage and Divorce*, Table 3-5, p. 46.

22. Ibid., Table 3-11. These figures are standardized for age.

23. U.S. Bureau of the Census, Current Population Reports, ser. P-20, no. 242, p. 3.

24. Alvin T. Onaka and David Yaukey, "Reproductive Time Lost Due to Marital Union Dissolution in San Jose, Costa Rica," forthcoming in *Population Studies,* probably November 1973.

Chapter 6
Cohort Marital Status and
First Marriage

1. Chapter 2.

2. Two demographers usually credited with pioneering the development of nuptiality tables have been Wilson H. Grabill, "Attrition Life Table for the Single Population," *Journal of the American Statistical Association* 40 (September 1945): 364-75, and Walter Mertens, "Methodological Aspects of the Construction of Nuptiality Tables," *Demography*, 2 (1965): 317-48.

3. Coale, "Age Patterns of Marriage."

4. United Nations, *Manual III: Methods of Population Projections by Sex and Age* (New York: United Nations, 1956), pp. 42-44.

5. Coale, "Age Patterns of Marriage," p. 203.

6. Ibid., p. 204.

Chapter 7
Implications for a
Fertility-Reduction Policy

1. Chapter 2.

2. Chapter 5.

3. Chapter 6.

4. Ansley J. Coale, "Age Patterns of Marriage," *Population Studies* 21 (July 1971): 193-214.

5. Chapter 2.

6. For a very recent treatment of the issues raised here, see June Sklar, "Marriage Regulation and the California Birth Rate," in Kingsley Davis and Frederick M. Styles (eds.), *California's Twenty Million: Research Contributions to Population Policy* (Population Monographs Series, no. 10; Berkeley: University of California, 1971), pp. 165-206.

7. A stimulating recent essay on this general topic is Kingsley Davis, "The Nature and Purpose of Population Policy," in Davis and Styles, *California's Twenty Million*, pp. 3-29.

Index

Index

113

About the Author

David Yaukey is Professor of Sociology at the University of Massachusetts, Amherst and currently is Director of the Social and Demographic Research Institute there. He has worked abroad in several cultures, teaching at the American University of Beirut in Lebanon, serving as Field Associate for the Population Council in Bangladesh, and visiting for one year the United Nations Centro Latinoamericano de Demografia in Santiago, Chile. His initial book was *Fertility Differences in a Modernizing Country: A Survey of Lebanese Couples*, published by Princeton University Press in 1961. Since that time his professional interest in fertility has persisted and resulted in numerous articles and research reports. Recently that interest has been complemented by one in nuptiality, exemplified by the present book.